Creating Successful Dementia Care Settings

Volume 2

Maximizing Cognitive and Functional Abilities

The complete set of books in
Creating Successful Dementia Care Settings
includes

Volume 1: **Understanding the Environment Through Aging Senses**
Volume 2: **Maximizing Cognitive and Functional Abilities**
Volume 3: **Minimizing Disruptive Behaviors**
Volume 4: **Enhancing Identity and Sense of Home**

Training videos for
Creating Successful Dementia Care Settings
include

Maximizing Cognitive and Functional Abilities (companion to Volume 2)
Minimizing Disruptive Behaviors (companion to Volume 3)
Enhancing Self and Sense of Home (companion to Volume 4)
(See ordering information at end of book.)

Creating Successful Dementia Care Settings

Developed by Margaret P. Calkins, M.Arch., Ph.D.

Volume 2
Maximizing Cognitive and Functional Abilities

Volume Authors
Sherylyn H. Briller, Ph.D.,
Mark A. Proffitt, M.Arch.,
Kristin Perez, OTR/L,
Margaret P. Calkins, M.Arch., Ph.D.,
and John P. Marsden, M.Arch., Ph.D.

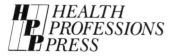
HEALTH
PROFESSIONS
PRESS

Baltimore • London • Winnipeg • Sydney

Health Professions Press, Inc.
Post Office Box 10624
Baltimore, Maryland 21285-0624

www.healthpropress.com

Typeset by Barton Matheson Willse & Worthington, Baltimore, Maryland.
Printed in the United States of America by Versa Press, Inc., East Peoria, Illinois.
Interior illustrations by David Fedan.

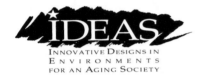

INNOVATIVE DESIGNS IN
ENVIRONMENTS
FOR AN AGING SOCIETY

Margaret P. Calkins, M.Arch., Ph.D., is president of I.D.E.A.S. (Innovative Designs in Environments for an Aging Society), Inc., a consultation, education, and research firm dedicated to exploring the therapeutic potential of the environment as it relates to older adults who are frail and impaired. I.D.E.A.S., Inc., is based in Kirtland, Ohio.

The case examples in this book series are based on the authors' actual experiences. In all instances, names and identifying details have been changed to protect confidentiality.

Library of Congress Cataloging-in-Publication Data

Calkins, Margaret P.
    Creating successful dementia care settings / developed by Margaret P. Calkins.
        p.   cm.
    Includes bibliographical references and index.
    Contents: Vol. 1. Understanding the environment through aging senses—v. 2. Maximizing cognitive and functional abilities—v. 3. Minimizing disruptive behaviors—v. 4. Enhancing identity and sense of home.
        ISBN 1-878812-72-6 (v. 1)—ISBN 1-878812-73-4 (v. 2)—ISBN 1-878812-74-2 (v. 3)—ISBN 1-878812-75-0 (v. 4)
        1. Dementia—Patients—Care. 2. Dementia—Patients—Long-term care. 3. Health facilities—Administration. I. Title.

RC521.C35 2001
362.1'9683—dc21   2001039141

British Cataloguing in Publication Data are available from the British Library.

Series
Contents

About the Authors xiii
Acknowledgments xv
Preface xvii
User's Guide xix

Volume 1

Chapter 1   **The Senses** 1
             Sensory Stimulation 2
Chapter 2   **Vision** 5
             How Vision Changes with Age 5
             What Staff Can Do 9
                 Before Personal Care
                 Keeping Residents Active
             What the Environment Can Do 11
                 Lighting
                 Ways to Improve Poor or Inadequate Lighting
                 Color and Pattern
                 Room Features
Chapter 3   **Hearing** 25
             How Hearing Changes with Age .25
             What Staff Can Do 26
                 Communication Techniques
                 Socialization
             What the Environment Can Do 28
                 Excess Noise
                 Acoustical Treatments for Hard Surfaces
Chapter 4   **Smell and Taste** 33
             How Smell and Taste Change with Age 33
             What Staff Can Do 34
                 Incorporating Positive Smells and Tastes
                 Using Smells with Personal Meaning
                 Minimizing Negative Smells
             What the Environment Can Do 36
                 Reducing Negative Odors
                 Using Positive Smells and Tastes as Room Cues
                 Using Aromatherapy
                 Planting Therapeutic Gardens

Chapter 5 **Touch** 41
How Touch Changes with Age 41
What Staff Can Do 42
  Incorporating Touch into Therapeutic Activities
  When Touch Is Not Appropriate
What the Environment Can Do 44
  Improving the Textural Environment
  Avoiding Abrasive Elements
  Regulating Temperature
Bibliography 49
Index 51

Volume 2

Chapter 1 **What Are Functional Abilities?** 1
Functional Abilities in Older People .2
  A Myth About Aging
  When Functional Abilities Become a Problem
    at Home
  Moving into Long-Term Care Facilities
  What Is Excess Disability?
Functional Abilities in Older People with Dementia 4
  Physical Factors
  Cognitive Factors
  Social Factors
  Environmental Factors
Assessment as a Multidimensional Process 7
  Assessment of Physical Factors
  Assessment of Cognitive Factors
  Assessment of Social Factors
  Assessment of Environmental Factors

Chapter 2 **Orientation** 11
What Staff Can Do 15
  Orientation to Time
  Orientation to Place
  Reality Orientation Versus Validation
What the Environment Can Do 18
  Spatial Adjacencies
  Cueing
  Rooms
Where to Find Products 38

Chapter 3 **Mobility** 43
Mobility in Older People 43
  Psychological Issues
  Physiological Issues
  Falls

Mobility in Older People with Dementia 49
   Apraxia
   Risk of Falling in Residents with Dementia
   Restraints
What Staff Can Do 53
   Contributors to Resident Falls
   When Mobility Becomes Significantly Impaired
   The Truth About Restraints
   Mobility Aids
   Exercise to Promote and Maintain Physical
     Conditioning
   Difference Staff Can Make in Successful
     Rehabilitation
What the Environment Can Do 68
   Environmental Aspects that Support Mobility
   Improving Mobility in Specific Areas
   Flooring
   Furniture
   Handrails
   Communication Devices
   Residents' Rooms and Public Areas
Where to Find Products 83

Chapter 4   **Continence** 91
Incontinence as a Part of Normal Aging 91
   Incontinence Compounded by Dementia
Changes in a Resident's Continence 92
What Staff Can Do 93
   Interventions
   Reducing Embarrassment When Assistance Is Needed
What the Environment Can Do 96
   Finding the Bathroom
   Finding the Toilet
   Transferring to and from the Toilet
Where to Find Products 100

Chapter 5   **Eating** 103
How Eating Changes with Age 104
   Social Issues
   Physical Issues
How Dementia Affects the Experience of Eating 106
   Memory Problems
   Problems with Chewing and Swallowing
   When Residents Are No Longer Able to Eat
What Staff Can Do 110
   Reasons that Residents May Reject Food
   Creating a Therapeutic Setting for Dining
   Administrative Support
   Interventions to Improve Eating

	What the Environment Can Do 121
	Finding the Dining Room
	Minimizing Excess Disability
	Where to Find Products 134
Chapter 6	**Dressing** 143
	When Older Adults Have Trouble Dressing 143
	Physical Issues 144
	Difficulties of Dressing for Residents with Dementia 145
	What Staff Can Do 145
	Understanding Residents' Feelings
	Taking a Therapeutic Approach
	Stages of Dressing
	How It Feels to Need Help Getting Dressed
	What the Environment Can Do 157
	Closet/Wardrobe Modification
	Recognizing the Contents of Closets
	Closet and Room Lighting
	Grooming Center
	Where to Find Products 162
Chapter 7	**Bathing** 167
	How Important Is Bathing? 167
	Why Do Some Residents Dislike Bathing? 168
	How Often Should Residents Bathe? 168
	What Staff Can Do 169
	Undressing Residents
	Privacy
	Running Water
	Air and Water Temperatures
	What the Environment Can Do 172
	Using a Tub that Fits Residents' Needs
	Privacy Issues
	Controlling Air and Water Temperatures
	Creating Pleasant Tub Rooms
	Where to Find Products 177
Bibliography 183	
Index 189	

Volume 3

Chapter 1	**What Is Disruptive Behavior?** 1
	Past Responses to Disruptive Behaviors 2
	Why Do These Behaviors Occur? .4
	Agenda Behavior Approach
	Using a Behavior Tracking Process
Chapter 2	**Wandering** 9
	What Is Wandering? 9
	Motivators for Wandering 11

Past Responses to Wandering 12
Strategies to Address Wandering 13
What Staff Can Do 15
    Inhibitors to Social Involvement
    Promoting Social Involvement
    Orientation
    Excessive Walking
What the Environment Can Do 21
    Promoting Social Interaction and Diversion
    Orientation to Place
    Limiting Wandering into Nonresidential/Private
      Areas
    Excessive Walking
Where to Find Products 30

Chapter 3   **Attempting to Leave** 39
Why Residents Might Want to Leave 39
Patterns of Leaving 40
Determining Appropriate Interventions 41
What Staff Can Do 42
    Addressing Patterns of Exiting
    Methods for Decreasing Exiting
    When a Resident Successfully Leaves a Unit
What the Environment Can Do 45
    Minimizing Confinement and Regulating Stimulation
    Modifying Doorways to Reduce Exiting
    Security Systems
    Elevators as Specific Problem Areas
    Windows as Specific Problem Areas
Where to Find Products 58

Chapter 4   **Rummaging and Hoarding** 65
Common Reasons for Rummaging 66
Common Reasons for Hoarding 67
What Staff Can Do 68
    Creating Places to Rummage
    Increasing Sensory Stimulation
    Providing Opportunities to Be Productive
What the Environment Can Do 70
    Creating Places to Rummage
    Creating Places of Productivity
    Returning the Idea of Control
Where to Find Products 72

Chapter 5   **Combative Behaviors** 75
How Problematic Are Combative Behaviors? 76
Causes of Combative Behaviors 77
    Physiological Issues
    Emotional Issues
    Environmental Issues

Addressing Combative Behaviors 80
    Identifying the Causes
    Using Restraints
    Agitation as a Precursor
What Staff Can Do 82
    Staff Training
    Approaches to Use During Personal Care
    Interventions for Overstimulation
    Intervening in a Combative Situation
What the Environment Can Do 88
    Addressing Combative Behaviors During Bathing
    Addressing Environmental Auditory and Visual
      Causes of Stress
Where to Find Products 97

Chapter 6   **Socially Inappropriate Behaviors** 105
Disruptive Vocalizations 105
    Contributing Factors
    Assessing Behavior
    Discussing the Behavior with Direct Care Staff
Inappropriate Sexual Behaviors 107
    Resident Sexuality
    Underlying Causes
Repetitive Behaviors 110
What Staff Can Do 111
    Disruptive Vocalizations
    Sexual Behaviors
    Repetitive Behaviors

Bibliography 123
Appendix A: Behavior Tracking Form 127
Appendix B: Sensory Stimulation Assessment 131
Index 135

Volume 4

Chapter 1   **Overview of Home-Based Philosophy of Care** 1
Models of Care 2
    Medical Model
    Residential Model
    Hospitality Model
Conclusion 6

Chapter 2   **Personalization** 7
Expressing the Self 7
Understanding the Self 9
Marking a Territory as Your Own .9
How Personalization Changes with Age and Relocation 10
    Preserving the Self
    Relocation

How Dementia Affects Personalization 14
What Staff Can Do 16
    Developing Policies to Encourage Personalization
    Helping Residents with Personalization
What the Environment Can Do 21
    Residents' Bedrooms
    Private Bathrooms
    Bedroom Entryways
    Exterior Window Treatments
    Interior Shared Spaces
    Tub Room
    Outdoor Shared Spaces
Where to Find Products 33

Chapter 3   **Roles and Activities** 39
Definition of Self 40
Well-Being 41
How Roles and Activities Change with Age and Relocation . . .43
    Loss of Roles and Activities
    New Roles and Activities
    Role Confusion
    Relocation
How Dementia Affects Roles and Activities 47
What Staff Can Do 48
    Providing Appropriate Activities
    Making the Activities Work
What the Environment Can Do 57
    Domestic Activities
    Work Activities
    Leisure Activities
Where to Find Products 65

Chapter 4   **Privacy** 71
Letting Your Hair Down 71
Self-Reflection 73
Control 73
Protecting Information About the Self 74
How Privacy Needs Change with Age and Relocation 76
    Decreased Social Support
    Health Problems
    Relocation
How Dementia Affects Privacy 79
What Staff Can Do 80
    Develop Policies to Protect Privacy
    Recognize Residents' Privacy Needs
What the Environment Can Do 85
    Shared Residents' Bedrooms
    Residents' Bathrooms
    Hallways

Indoor Shared Spaces
Outdoor Shared Spaces
Where to Find Products 90
Chapter 5   **Autonomy and Control** 93
Choice 94
Well-Being 95
How Autonomy and Control Change with Age and
        Relocation 97
        Social and Physical Losses
        Relocation
How Dementia Affects Autonomy and Control 100
What Staff Can Do 101
        Developing Policies to Encourage Control
        Providing Meaningful Choices
What the Environment Can Do 107
        Private Areas
        Choices
        Orientation Cues
        Access to the Outdoors
        Activity Choices
Where to Find Products 111
Chapter 6   **Residential Design** 115
What the Environment Can Do 116
        Spatial Adjacencies
        Scale
        Purpose-Specific Rooms
        Decor
Where to Find Products 134
Bibliography 143
Appendix A: Resident's Social History 147
Appendix B: Hanging Pictures and Artwork .161
Appendix C: Toxicity of Common House and Garden Plants 163
Index 171

About
the
Authors

Margaret P. Calkins, M.Arch., Ph.D., is President of I.D.E.A.S. Inc. (Innovative Designs in Environments for an Aging Society), a consultation, education, and research firm dedicated to exploring the therapeutic potential of the environment—social and organizational as well as physical—particularly as it relates to older adults who are frail and impaired. She is also Senior Fellow Emeritus of the Institute on Aging and Environment at the University of Wisconsin-Milwaukee.

Dr. Calkins holds degrees in both psychology and architecture. A member of several national organizations and panels that focus on issues of care for older adults with cognitive impairment, she speaks frequently at conferences nationally and internationally. She has published extensively, and her book *Design for Dementia: Planning Environments for the Elderly and the Confused* (National Health Publication, 1998) was the first comprehensive design guide for special care units for people with dementia.

Dr. Calkins is Director and a founding member of SAGE (Society for the Advancement of Gerontological Environments), and has been a juror for numerous design competitions.

Sherylyn H. Briller, Ph.D., is Assistant Professor of Anthropology at Wayne State University. She is a medical anthropologist who specializes in aging research. Dr. Briller received her master's and doctorate degrees and a graduate certificate in gerontology from Case Western Reserve University. She has been actively involved in the field of aging for more than a decade, both domestically and abroad. Her diverse career has included working as an activities coordinator in a skilled nursing facility, a program director at a community senior center, and a gerontological researcher in the United States of America and Asia. Her long-term care expertise includes philosophy/model of care, staff training, activity programming, and ethnic/cultural issues relating to aging. She has consulted, published, and given presentations to numerous audiences including policy makers, researchers, administrators, direct caregivers, and consumers.

John P. Marsden, M.Arch., Ph.D., is an assistant professor in the College of Design, Construction and Planning and a core faculty member of the Institute on Aging at the University of Florida. He holds degrees in architecture from Carnegie Mellon University, the University of Arizona, and the University of Michigan. Dr. Marsden has worked for several architecture firms, was an associate at I.D.E.A.S., Inc., and has consulted with designers and long-term care administrators. He is a frequent speaker at gerontology and environmental design conferences and served as a juror for the 1999 Best of Seniors' Housing Awards, sponsored by the National Council on Seniors' Housing, a division of the National Association of Home Builders.

Kristin Perez, OTR/L, received her bachelor's degree in gerontology from Bowling Green State University and a certificate in occupational therapy from Cleveland State University. Ms. Perez has experience in direct care, programming, management, and research in dementia care settings. She has assisted older adults in maximizing their level of independence and life satisfaction in assisted living, nursing facility, adult day services, and hospital settings. Ms. Perez has been actively involved in numerous research projects addressing dementia care practices and environments, including project management. She has also provided consultation to long-term care facilities regarding dementia care practices and environmental influences.

Mark A. Proffitt, M.Arch., is an architectural researcher with Dorsky Hodgson + Partners, an architectural firm that specializes in designs for older adults. His primary responsibilities include post-occupancy evaluations of completed projects and the programming protocol for the elderly design studio. He strongly believes that good design must build on research. Mr. Proffitt received his master's degree in architecture from the University of Wisconsin–Milwaukee, where he was a fellow with the Institute on Aging and Environment. After receiving his degree, he served as a facilities architect and manager for a developer of retirement communities. Mr. Proffitt has also co-authored a book on the creation and evaluation of an innovative health center and has spoken at several industry-related conferences.

Acknowledgments

Creative endeavors are nurtured to fruition by the ideas and efforts of myriad people at every step of a process. While the original conceptualization for the project was spearheaded by Maggie Calkins, with input from Jerry Weisman, this was very much a team project. All of the authors' talents and contributions were integral and critical to the evolution of the larger project from which these volumes are drawn. In addition, Eileen Lipstreuer, Chari Weber, and Rebecca Meehan deserve as much credit for their contributions to the project as the names that appear on the title pages of these volumes. The videos that accompany these volumes are a direct result of their industriousness. Thanks also to Jesse Epstein, of Cinecraft, and David Litz, the videographer, and to David Fedan for his charming illustrations.

Much of the project was funded by the National Institute on Aging (grant R44 AG12311) and enthusiastically supported and championed by Marcia Ory. We were also fortunate to have a team of nationally recognized experts whose input—both conceptual and practical—was invaluable. We extend our gratitude to Powell Lawton, Jerry Weisman, Phil Sloane, Joe Foley, Susan Gilster, Kitty Buckwalter, Jeanne Teresi, Doug Holmes, and Sheryl Zimmerman. Peter Whitehouse, Elisabeth Koss, Clive Gilmore, and Monte Levinson shared their keen intellect and significant insight with us as we started this project. During the most stressful periods of the project, Cassie and Ted always seemed to come to our rescue.

We would like to thank the numerous individuals whose publications and conference presentations enriched our understanding of the complex nature of dementia, and provided myriad ideas for creative solutions to difficult challenges. We also appreciate the endless hours of listening and thoughtful contributions of the many family, friends, and colleagues who helped out in so many ways as the project evolved over 4 years. To the numerous facility staff and administrators who listened to, read, questioned, and critiqued our efforts and dialogued with us about them, it was for you that we embarked on this voyage. We are pleased to share what we have learned with you.

Preface

All too often, we see well-intentioned caregivers unnecessarily limit or downplay the potential remaining abilities of the older adults with dementia for whom they care. Caregivers seem to assume that because a person has dementia, every behavior and every expression of anxiety, fear, or anger is a direct consequence of the dementing illness. And, because dementia impairs care recipients' cognitive abilities, many caregivers believe that they have the right and the responsibility to make all decisions for those they care for.

It has been the authors' experience that the factors that affect the behavior of residents with dementia are complex. Our approach to understanding their behavior focuses on the person, on his or her typical needs and desires, on the limitations imposed by age-related changes, and on the effects of aspects of the environment.

Our fundamental philosophy is that we must first consider those in our care as people, who have many of the same needs, desires, and wishes as anyone else. To lose the ability to make decisions that affect virtually every aspect of living is devastating. To have that ability further eroded by care providers and care settings that eliminate almost every opportunity for choice and control is unacceptable.

It is the authors' hope that in using the information contained within *Creating Successful Dementia Care Settings*, facilities will create meaningful care settings by educating and sensitizing staff and by making full use of the environmental resources available to them.

User's Guide

The authors' goal in writing this four-volume series was to create an easy-to-use reference to help care providers understand and more appropriately manage, through the environment, the broad array of behaviors and changing abilities that occur with dementia. One must first recognize the importance of accommodating the basic needs of all people, and then one must consider that most people with dementia are older and, therefore, experience the world through sensory modalities that are changing or that have been altered by aging. Vision, hearing, touch, taste, and smell all change with age, and sensory changes often affect behavior. For example, it may not be dementia but simply poor vision that hinders a person's ability to read signs or an activity calendar. Volume 1, *Understanding the Environment Through Aging Senses* helps caregivers to be more sensitive to how these sensory changes can affect a person's basic functioning.

Only after the needs of the resident as a person like anyone else and as an older person with changing sensory experiences have been acknowledged can one consider the unique needs of the individual as an older person with dementia. There is no denying that the neuropathological changes that occur in the brain of a person with dementia affect his or her ability to perceive, make sense of, and operate effectively in the surrounding environment. Basic tasks, such as dressing and eating, that once were easy become increasingly difficult. The inability to interpret what someone is saying, to identify faces or objects, or to understand his or her current location can easily lead to fear and resistance to care. Volumes 2 and 3, *Maximizing Cognitive and Functional Abilities* and *Minimizing Disruptive Behaviors*, respectively, focus on these issues.

Enhancing Identity and Sense of Home, Volume 4, addresses issues that are primarily related to basic human needs such as privacy, autonomy, identity, and personal space. Much of the information is appropriate not only for people with dementia but also for cognitively alert individuals in long-term care settings.

The more that you, as a caregiver, understand all of the factors that affect the person or people whose care is entrusted to you, the better able you are to see the world as they do. Thus, the beginning of each chapter in all of the volumes presents the individual topic from the residents' perspective, including contributing factors and influences on specific behaviors or issues. In addition, these sections offer ideas for assessing problems and implementing interventions. This level of information is particularly useful for staff members who manage and/or train direct care staff. The authors hope that this information will broaden staff's knowledge on the topic and that they will pass the information along to others who care for residents.

The residents' perspective section is followed by "What Staff Can Do," which provides information on social interactions between staff and residents and ideas for structured and spontaneous activities on the unit. Some interventions focus on teaching direct care staff to take a different approach to particular situations, whereas other interventions are provided for staff who plan structured activities and programs.

The third main section of each chapter, "What the Environment Can Do," offers suggestions for modifications or changes that can be made to the physical environment so that your facility becomes more supportive of the residents, particularly those with dementia. Many of the suggested changes cost nothing and involve only a different use of the environment or a small modification using materials you probably already have on hand. Other changes are low in cost, requiring the purchase of a few additional products or materials. Finally, if your facility is able to upgrade or replace some of its furnishings or equipment, we have provided practical advice in "What the Environment Can Do" on what to consider when purchasing a product. Many of the modifications suggested in this section explain how these modifications benefit the residents and the staff who care for them.

The final section of each chapter, "Where to Find Products," lists specific manufacturers and distributors of the products mentioned in the text. There is some repetition in these sections across the four volumes so that you do not have to refer to a separate volume for the information. Many of the manufacturers and catalogs also carry more products than those highlighted in our lists. This section is followed by a summary sheet, which boils down the chapter text into an easy-to-remember, quick overview. We have also provided an area for you to make notes about your own staff and facility. Managerial staff may wish to use the summary sheets as handouts to accompany direct care staff training, or to post them by the time clock or nurses' station or include them in staff's pay envelopes. All staff, including business office, social services, dietary, and housekeeping, may appreciate this quick overview of issues because they likely interact with residents daily.

At the conclusion of each volume, a detailed bibliography and suggested readings help you learn more about issues in the individual volumes. The Behavior Tracking Form and Sensory Stimulation Assessment appendixes appear at the end of Volume 3. Staff can use these forms to examine the occurrence of behaviors and aspects of the environment more closely. Each blank form is accompanied by explanatory information and a sample completed form. Volume 4 includes three appendixes, all designed to help residents feel more at home in the facility and to protect their safety.

In addition to the four volumes, there are three videotapes that relate to Volumes 2–4. They were designed to be staff education resources and provide an additional way of helping all staff learn how to create successful dementia care settings (see ordering information at the end of each volume).

We at I.D.E.A.S., Inc., wish you success in developing a high-quality environment for caregiving. It is our hope that facilities will use this information to create meaningful dementia care settings by educating and sensitizing staff. If you are having a hard time determining which aspects of your care setting most need to be changed or modified, we hope that you will contact us directly (440-256-1880 or info@IDEASconsultingInc.com).

1
What Are Functional Abilities?

All people like to feel as if they do things well. From childhood, we are praised for our accomplishments—dressing independently, tying our own shoes, riding a bicycle, and going to school. As we get older, we continue to learn to do more complex things such as reading, driving, and managing a checkbook. Most adults pride themselves on being able to perform these activities independently.

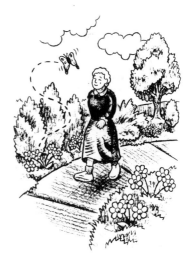

Functional abilities are the physical and cognitive skills that enable people to perform routine tasks independently. They are the skills that are required for activities of daily living (ADLs), such as dressing, eating, and bathing, and independent activities of daily living (IADLs), including shopping, handling money, and managing one's affairs. We rarely think about what it takes to do these routine activities unless problems develop. For example, when someone is under a great deal of stress, such as when a family member is ill or there are problems at work, he or she may become easily distracted and make mistakes that would not normally be made. These mistakes could include depositing checks without endorsing them or locking the keys in the car. When these types of problems occur, we may feel frustrated and angry with ourselves, but usually these feelings pass quickly. Depending on the circumstances, these mishaps may even become funny stories that can be told later.

When problems with functional abilities occur regularly however, it may no longer seem like a laughing matter. Instead, we may become quite alarmed about the situation. Not being able to perform everyday activities is upsetting to people who have been used to doing these tasks independently for many years. Having problems with functional abilities often negatively affects their sense of personal worth and self-confidence and may even make them feel like total failures. Because it is embarrassing to admit these kinds of problems to others, people may suffer in silence and feel depressed. Sometimes they may even stop doing their regular activities such as getting dressed, going out, and socializing with others. Thus, problems with functional abilities can diminish quality of life when these difficulties occur over time.

FUNCTIONAL ABILITIES IN OLDER PEOPLE

With advancing age, people often experience increasing problems with functional abilities. It has been predicted that the number of people older than age 65 will double and the number of people 85 years old and older will triple between the years 1989 and 2030 (Emlet, Crabtree, Condon, & Treml, 1996). Therefore, it is important to understand how age-related changes affect functional abilities. With this knowledge, you will be better able to consider ways to help older people maximize their remaining abilities and create supportive environments that enable them to do this.

A Myth About Aging

In our culture, a common belief is that old age is a period of steady decline and it is not possible to maintain or improve physical and mental function later in life. However, a great deal of research (e.g., Birren & Schaie, 1990) has shown that this does not have to be the case. A therapeutic approach that emphasizes thinking about the potential of older adults rather than just their limitations is preferable. We should think about what older people can do and what it would take for them to be able to function more independently rather than automatically doing things for them.

There are many reasons why we may try to do things for older people rather than help them to do these things independently. We may be trying

- To be respectful or helpful
- To repay older people for all that they have done for us
- To save time and do things more efficiently

Although these all are logical reasons for doing things for older people, they do not necessarily take into account what older people may or may not want us to do for them. Consider the following example.

Leona invited her mother for dinner but, rather than letting her help in the kitchen, encouraged her to sit in the living room like a guest. Although Leona was doing this because her mom had worked so hard for so many years, Leona's mother assumed that it was because her arthritis makes it hard for her to do kitchen tasks such as opening jars and peeling potatoes. She actually would have been happier helping out and felt badly because she was not asked. Leona came into the living room to find her mother crying on the sofa. After she told Leona why she was crying, Leona invited her to come into the kitchen to help prepare the rest of the meal. The next day Leona made plans to go out and buy some easy-to-grip utensils so that her mother could work more easily in the kitchen.

This example illustrates several important points. First, problems with functional abilities can include physical, mental, social, and environmental components. Second, making relatively small changes in the way in which things are done (e.g., using adaptive tools) can make a big difference in the lives of older people who are trying to remain independent. Third, the self-image and sense of self-worth of older people can be affected deeply by these difficulties. Throughout this volume, consideration is given to how these problems overlap and influence what older people can do.

When Functional Abilities Become a Problem at Home

For many older people living in the community, noticing their functional abilities diminish is frightening because it may be a sign that they will not be able to continue to live independently. They may try to get along doing the best that they can, but sometimes the situation may become too much for them to handle. Families often become aware of these problems when crises arise (e.g., older people stop paying bills, burn themselves while cooking, fall while going to the basement). These problems may occur for a variety of reasons, including increased physical frailty, poor vision, and short-term memory deficits. At this point, families may become alarmed and insist that their older loved ones move into more supportive settings where they will receive more assistance.

Moving into Long-Term Care Facilities

Sometimes decisions to move into long-term care facilities are made jointly by the older person and family members, and sometimes they are not. Some older people may feel tremendous relief to be living in an environment in which help is always available; others may be extremely depressed at having to leave their own homes. Moving into a new, unfamiliar environment can be especially challenging for older people who already have difficulties with functional abilities. When they cannot see well, it may be hard to read the signs in the facility telling them where rooms or services are located. When they cannot hear well, they may not understand what staff are saying when they ask for directions. When they are depressed, they may not even want to perform basic tasks such as dressing and eating meals. These problems can make the transition to living in a new environment even harder.

What Is Excess Disability?

Excess disability exists when residents function at levels that are lower than their abilities indicate. Various physiological, cognitive, social, and environmental factors can contribute to excess disability, including fatigue; changes in caregiver, routine, or environment; excess or inappropriate stimulation; and physical problems such as pain or side effects of medications (Hall, 1994). Excess disability can be reversed if steps are taken to enable people to function at a higher level again. Minimizing excess disability should always be a priority because it supports the remaining abilities of residents and helps with preserving their dignity.

FUNCTIONAL ABILITIES
IN OLDER PEOPLE WITH DEMENTIA

Residents with dementia often experience significant problems with functional abilities. As is the case with older people in general, these problems are often the result of a combination of physical, cognitive, social, and environmental factors. This section considers briefly what impact each of these factors has on older people with dementia.

Physical Factors

Physical factors are one of the most important reasons why residents with dementia have functional disabilities. These problems can result from both age- and disease-related components. For example, impairments in the following physical systems can affect function (Chandler & Duncan, 1993; Guccione, 1993):

- Musculoskeletal system (e.g., limited range of motion)
- Neuromuscular system (e.g., muscle weakness)
- Cardiopulmonary system (e.g., decreased lung capacity)
- Sensory system (e.g., poor vision or hearing)
- Integumentary system (e.g., pressure sores)
- Mental state (e.g., confusion)

In particular, sensory losses can make it difficult for residents with dementia to perform ADLs. Most of these activities require using multiple senses together. Although sensory losses are challenging for all older people, they are especially problematic for people with dementia. Volume 1 in this series examines how functional skills are integrally linked to sensory perception. Understanding how they are linked will enable staff to take a more holistic approach in considering how to minimize excess disability in residents with multiple types of problems.

Cognitive Factors

Cognitive factors also affect the ability of residents with dementia to perform ADLs. Reasons for changes in a particular resident's cognitive status include psychosocial issues (e.g., depression), drug interactions or overmedication, infections, and nutritional and metabolic imbalances (Emlet et al., 1996). In particular, residents with dementia often have a variety of problems, including trouble with

- Remembering recent events
- Recognizing places, things, or people
- Following instructions
- Executing a sequence of actions

Apraxia

Residents with dementia frequently have apraxia, a neurological condition that causes them to have difficulty with order or sequence. For example, these residents typically have problems remembering how to perform the steps of routine motor tasks such as walking and eating. Apraxia can cause tremendous problems with ADLs such as dressing. Clothing may be put on oddly, with clothes inside out, backward, or on the wrong body part. Having problems with sequence or order may also make it difficult for a person to find his or her way in familiar places. Learning new patterns or sequences (e.g., the way to one's bedroom after a move to a long-term care facility) may be extremely difficult.

Agnosia

Another common problem among residents with dementia is agnosia, or trouble with recognizing or telling things apart. This problem can greatly affect people's ability to recognize familiar environmental objects and places. If the trouble is with objects, then the person may not be able to distinguish among a knife, a fork, and a spoon at mealtimes. Similarly, he or she may void in a wastebasket rather than in a toilet because the objects look quite similar, because he or she is confused about the purpose of the object, or for both reasons. The combination of agnosia and either low vision or poor hearing also can worsen people's difficulties with functional abilities.

Aphasia

Communicating with residents with dementia can be quite a challenge. These residents often suffer from aphasia, or trouble finding words to express thoughts or making sense out of words that are spoken by someone else. Trouble with speaking is called *expressive aphasia*. Expressive aphasia can be minor, such as having a word on the tip of the tongue but not being able to say it, or it can be severe, with words or sounds mixed so that what is said is nonsensical.

It is important to remember that mixed-up words may not mean mixed-up thinking. A person may be able to think quite clearly but not be able to put those thoughts into the right words. It is also possible for a person who thinks quite clearly to have trouble following words that are spoken. Because this is highly embarrassing, the person may try to cover up by making comments or giving answers that could apply to anything. In some cases, residents with aphasia may understand bits and pieces of what is said, or speech may sound like a foreign language or nonsense to them. Therefore, it may be difficult for them to understand even simple instructions or cues that staff may give during ADLs.

Concentration

Residents with dementia commonly have problems with concentration and judgment. Not being able to filter out noises or activities around them can greatly affect their functional abilities. For example, if people are talking in the dining room, and there is the clatter of silverware and a radio playing, it may be hard for residents to tune out this noise and focus on eating. What we hear as background noise may be intense noise to them. Residents with dementia often have trouble concentrating when multiple things are going on at the same time.

Social Factors

People with dementia, especially in the early stage, often are aware of their losses in functional abilities. Feelings of depression, lack of self-esteem, isolation, anxiety, and grief commonly accompany these functional losses. Many times these residents may feel as though they are the only ones who experience these difficulties. It may be difficult for older people who are used to being independent and competent to accept some of the types of personal assistance that they may now require. Staff should be supportive and listen to these residents when they are frustrated. Some older people may believe that if they cannot do things the way they used to do them, they no longer want to do them at all. Although it is easy to understand why older adults may believe this, it is more therapeutic for them to continue to use their remaining abilities for as long as they can. The saying "use it or lose it" is definitely true when it comes to functional abilities.

Environmental Factors

The environment can either support or limit the functional abilities of residents with dementia. The design of specific features in the environment (e.g., lighting, handrails) can assist residents with physical limitations to get around more easily. However, it is equally important to consider how well residents with dementia can read or figure out cues in the environment to help them get where they want to go. It can be extremely tiring and frustrating for residents with dementia when the environment is not supportive and does not provide features that help them with wayfinding. The sections called "What the Environment Can Do" throughout this volume provide recommendations for how to make the environment more user-friendly.

ASSESSMENT AS A MULTIDIMENSIONAL PROCESS

Residents with dementia will not necessarily experience all of the problems already discussed. The degree to which functional abilities are affected also vary among individuals. Depending on the presence of other physical and sensory deficits and the level of support in the environment, residents with dementia may have more or less trouble with functional abilities. In general, as the dementia progresses, their functional abilities will be affected more and they will require more assistance. To maximize their remaining abilities, it is important to assess continually what these residents can do.

The overall goal of functional assessment should be to understand both clinical and nonclinical factors that may contribute to excess disability. Many good clinical resources are available for use in long-term care settings (e.g., Emlet et al., 1996; Gallo, 1995). A thorough assessment of functional status should take into account physical, cognitive, social, and environmental factors (Kane & Kane, 1981; Teresi, Lawton, Holmes, & Ory, 1997). Because residents with dementia often have communication problems, it can be difficult to assess their capabilities accurately. The conditions under which these residents are assessed may also greatly influence how they perform. A noisy clinic setting with the radio playing and conversations going on in the background may cause excess disability for residents with dementia. In this setting, they may be unable to hear or filter out the other things that may be going on around them and concentrate on the assessment.

Assessment of Physical Factors

One of the main goals of geriatric assessment has always been to determine the relationship between a person's physical impairments and his or her functional limitations (Treml, 1996). Physical and occupational therapists commonly collect information, including measurements of strength, range of motion, and coordination. Such information then is analyzed to determine whether the physical problem can be compensated for and, if so, what other steps need to be taken (e.g., modifying the environment, changing the way that the task is done).

When assessing older people, it is important to remember that they may have good and bad days, depending on how they are feeling physically. If the assessment is done on a rainy day, then an older person with arthritis in his or her hands may have trouble buttoning a shirt because of additional stiffness in the hands. On a different day he or she might be able to do the same task with fewer problems. However, if the assessment records that the person is unable to do this task and changes are made or assistance provided so that he or she is never asked to do it again, then this skill may be lost over time.

Assessment of Cognitive Factors

Accurate assessment of the cognitive status of residents with dementia can be difficult. Many of these residents have communication problems that are directly related to their dementia and influence whether they can follow instructions and ultimately perform certain tasks. What is less commonly known is that other factors often influence how residents with cognitive impairments perform during assessments. Emlet et al. (1996) suggested the following tips when interviewing older adults:

- Face them directly.
- Sit somewhat close to them.
- Do not cover your face with your hands or other objects.
- Slow down your rate of speech; use simple sentences.
- Eliminate background noise (e.g., radio, television, other conversations).
- Repeat important points in different words if they cannot hear/understand what you are saying.

All of these factors can affect how well residents with dementia perform during assessment procedures.

Assessment of Social Factors

Many of us have felt nervous answering questions at a doctor's office, especially when the conversation occurs in an examining room. Most people are not used to being asked a battery of questions or performing a series of tasks while someone else watches. This is a highly unfamiliar and stressful situation. When older people are aware that there may be problems in some of the areas being tested, it can make them even more uncomfortable.

It is important to remember that many older adults today have had less formal education and experience with tasks involving reading, counting, or both. They may feel nervous when being tested on such tasks, especially when the tasks are timed. This generation of older adults also was taught to respect authority figures (e.g., doctors), and they may feel intimidated when being tested in clinical settings. Thus, they may not do as well in part because they are uncomfortable during the assessment procedure and afraid of giving the wrong answers.

Assessment can be a subjective process. Even if a standardized assessment instrument is used, the interaction between the resident being assessed and the person administering the assessment can affect how well the resident performs. If Mr. Colibri cannot hear what he is being asked to do because the examiner's voice echoes in the room, then he may appear not to understand the directions or may act inappropriately simply because he is trying to guess what is wanted. Similarly, if English is not Mrs. Esposito's native language, then she may be embarrassed to admit that she has trouble understanding the instructions. Yet, by not asking to have them repeated, she may then perform poorly on the test.

Assessment of Environmental Factors

It is generally best to assess the functional status of residents in their own environment because that is where they will most often be using skills such as dressing, eating, and toileting. To the greatest extent possible, staff doing the assessment should think about how to remove barriers that may be causing excess disability, such as inadequate lighting or poor furniture arrangement. One excellent resource that addresses these issues in detail is the book *Designing for Alzheimer's Disease: Strategies for Creating Better Care Environments* (Brawley, 1997). The sections entitled "What the Environment Can Do" in this volume frequently draw on this reference as a starting point for discussion of these issues.

Also, when older people move into a long-term care environment, they typically take some time to become comfortable navigating their new setting. Certain problems such as low vision, short-term memory deficits, or mobility problems can make this adjustment even harder. Many of these older people lived in their own homes for many years and knew exactly where everything was located. In these familiar environments, they may have been able to compensate for vision loss, confusion, or increased frailty. It is not surprising that many falls occur shortly after older adults move into a long-term care facility: The environment is still unfamiliar to them, and they have trouble figuring out where the light switches are, where the furniture is placed, or where the doorway is located. Discussions about how to assess the effects of specific environmental features on the functional abilities of residents with dementia can be found throughout the volume.

2

Orientation

At some point in their lives, most people have experienced the feeling of "starting over" and the need to learn a new way of doing things. Imagine that you move to a different place for a new job. When you first get there, you may feel disoriented because you do not know many people. It may seem strange when your telephone does not ring even once all day. There also may be less structure to your day if you are not working yet. The time may seem to go by either fast or slow without the normal routine of going to work. What you do during the day may be different from your regular routine as you

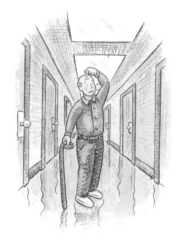

are forced to wait at home for furniture to arrive or utilities to be connected. Learning your way around in a new area also can be disconcerting because you are not yet familiar with landmarks that can help you orient yourself. This example illustrates why it may be disorienting to older adults to start a new life in a retirement community or long-term care center involving meeting new people, getting used to a new daily routine, and learning their way around a new environment.

Orientation refers to a person's awareness of his or her current situation and includes an awareness and understanding of people, time, and place. Orientation to people involves knowing who you are and recognizing other people—especially significant others such as a spouse or children. Orientation to time may include being aware of the year, month, season, day, and date. Orientation to place can be as broad as knowing the state or country in which you live or as specific as being able to find your bedroom.

Wayfinding is a process in which people use information in the environment to help them get to their desired destination. It refers to what people see, what they think about, and what they do to find their way from one location to another. Carpman (1991) identified five simple aspects of wayfinding:

1. Knowing where you are
2. Knowing what your destination is
3. Knowing (and following) the best route to your destination
4. Recognizing your destination on arrival
5. Finding your way back

One key issue in wayfinding is the ability to create a mental map to travel successfully from where you are to where you want to go. Being in a familiar setting helps with wayfinding because a person who has learned the way does not have to pay attention to all of the cues on every trip through the area. Some people also have a better sense of direction than others. They can learn quickly where everything is located in their new environment, whereas others may still become easily disoriented even after they have lived there for some time. When people regularly experience these difficulties, they often feel confused, embarrassed, and like an outsider. It is not surprising that people often find the time in which they are becoming oriented to a new setting to be somewhat tiring and stressful. This chapter discusses the reasons why older people, especially those moving into long-term care facilities, may experience problems with orientation and wayfinding.

Age-related sensory losses, short-term memory problems, or both often cause orientation problems in older people. For example, older people who cannot see well may not be able to read signs easily. Those who cannot hear well may have trouble understanding the directions they have requested. Those whose short-term memory is impaired may not remember the directions well even if they heard what was said.

Sometimes it may be hard to judge when an older person actually is experiencing orientation problems. Because older people have so many different experiences throughout their lives, it is not surprising that they have a difficult time remembering the names of all of the different pets that the family had or which winters had heavy storms. Such details tend to blur together when there is a lot to remember or certain events are not from the recent past. Older people with large families also may confuse the names of their various children and grandchildren. Although it makes sense that it may be hard to remember so much information, it may still be exceedingly frustrating to an older person when he or she is unable to remember the name of the 5-year-old granddaughter standing right in front of him or her, or is unable to see well enough to identify which grandchild is the one standing there.

It is often hard for others to watch a loved one develop orientation problems. Family and friends may have trouble knowing how to react appropriately to the changes that they are seeing. It is difficult to watch someone who always has been an exceptionally capable and intelligent person struggle to do routine activities of daily living (ADLs). Older people frequently are aware of the changes that are happening but feel powerless to do anything about them. The psychological distress caused by these kinds of problems can have serious physiological consequences for older people. Being upset often results in excess stress, an elevated heart rate, and elevated blood pressure. These physiological changes not only are detrimental to older people's physical health but also diminish their overall quality of life.

Orientation problems can make older people feel incompetent and not like themselves. Having these difficulties can produce so much anxiety that they may stop meeting new people or seeing the people they know, participating in new or routine activities, and going to different places or familiar places. When a spouse dies after many years of marriage, it can be hard for an older person to become oriented to his or her new life alone. The same is true when other important people, such as children, siblings, and close friends, either die or move away. These kinds of experiences can make older people realize how much their own identities were shaped by their relationships with others. It also may be difficult to orient to the changes in daily routines that inevitably occur.

Not doing all the things they used to do can make people feel lonely and isolated. Older people with orientation problems sometimes become so worried that they will not be able to remember what they were going to do at a particular time or where they were going to go on a particular day that they stop doing things completely. Whereas some older people may change their routine to simplify it, others may significantly reduce their activities and stop going out socially. Unfortunately, lack of interaction with other people may only add to their sense of disorientation.

Difficulties with finding one's way can be extremely stressful. Older adults often have trouble finding their way after they have moved from their own homes into a long-term care facility. At home, they probably knew where everything was, especially if they lived in the same house for many years. An environment that is less residential, is designed poorly, has confusing signage, and lacks cues often make it even harder for long-term care residents to find the places they want to go, especially for residents in a large, complex facility. Even on smaller units, some residents may experience significant difficulties in orientation and wayfinding. "What Staff Can Do" and "What the Environment Can Do" examine ways to minimize these problems.

In general, residents with dementia are prone to experiencing orientation problems. Residents with mild dementia, or sometimes even moderate dementia, may be aware of their problems but unable to avoid becoming confused. This can be depressing for them. Having dementia does not mean that one does not experience the same emotions as other people. Consequently, these residents still may be frustrated and embarrassed when they experience orientation difficulties.

One of the most disturbing aspects of dementia is the feeling of losing a sense of self. Orientation problems can contribute greatly to the feelings of fear, pain, and discomfort that accompany losing such an important piece of ourselves—our cognitive abilities. However, there is significant variation in what people's memories were like before the onset of dementia. Older people who have always had a poor memory for names and dates may not be as bothered by having memory problems because they have had such problems all of their lives. For others who prided themselves on their sharp memories, the development of memory problems can substantially affect their self-identities. They may develop ways to compensate for these problems by always writing down the names of new people they meet or making lists of what they intend to do that day. Yet this may not be enough to keep them from making mistakes, and they may feel frustrated that they can no longer remember things as they once were able to.

For residents with agnosia (trouble with recognizing or telling things apart), these problems may become even worse. If the trouble is with identifying faces, a resident with dementia may be unable to recognize a sister or daughter in a group of women. Similarly, the resident may remember that he or she is married but may not remember the face of his or her spouse. How would you feel if you went home after work and could no longer recognize the face of your spouse of 20 years?

Agnosia can interact with visuospatial dysfunction, causing residents to become easily disoriented and to have trouble judging where objects begin and end. Residents with dementia are also more likely to have trouble creating new mental maps of a unit and remembering routes that they have traveled even in the recent past. Therefore, the facility must pay special attention to providing enough information to help in the wayfinding process. (See "What the Environment Can Do" later in this chapter for a detailed discussion of the use of cues in the physical environment.)

For residents with dementia, problems with orientation may occur many times throughout the day. Difficulties with understanding or following a schedule can profoundly affect residents' feelings of autonomy, independence, and self-sufficiency. How would you feel if you made a date to meet someone in the lounge for coffee at 3 P.M. and you could not remember where the lounge was located? Worse yet, you might remember only that there was something that you were going to do that afternoon but not be sure what it was, and you might be too embarrassed to ask.

WHAT STAFF CAN DO

The frustration and loss of control that residents may feel when they have problems with orientation can be overwhelming, especially if these experiences are repeated many times throughout the day. What would it be like to be unable to recognize the faces of people around you—to see someone who looks like a stranger but insists he is your brother? What if you were to look in the mirror and found yourself wearing your bra on top of your blouse, to hear people talking all around you without your having the ability to focus on a conversation or to understand what someone is telling you, to have someone accuse you of using a wastebasket for a toilet, or to have no idea which way to turn to get to your bedroom? These kinds of situations are typical of the experiences of residents who have difficulties with orientation.

Orientation to Time

Residents with dementia may have trouble waiting patiently. For example, they may become agitated while seated at an empty table in the dining room when others are being served. Because their sense of time is distorted, minutes may feel like hours while they are waiting for food. Staff should find something for them to do while waiting; for example, offer them a beverage or a piece of bread to eat before their food is served. If certain residents have more trouble waiting than others, then make sure that they either are served first or come to the dining room after others have been served.

Orientation to Place

Residents who experience difficulty with orientation and wayfinding are more likely to become socially withdrawn unless staff help them to remain active. In addition to letting residents know the time and location of activity programs, staff can provide multiple sensory cues to attract them to where the fun is happening (e.g., smell of bread baking at mealtimes, certain music playing before a sing-along). Offering these types of cues can both maximize the remaining functional abilities of residents and make the jobs of staff easier.

The goal of a good cueing system is to minimize the frequency with which staff, family, or volunteers have to physically lead residents to specific locations. Nobody likes to feel lost, and it is embarrassing to ask continually for directions. In addition, the disorientation experienced by residents with dementia is worsened by sensory deficits. For example, research has shown that people with low vision have to make more and a greater variety of environmental decisions to get where they want to go (Passini & Proulx, 1988). Residents with low vision who also have dementia will have difficulty planning their journeys because they have trouble remembering details.

Familiar landmarks along the path they need to travel can assist residents with dementia to get where they want to go (e.g., the grandfather clock next to the dining room). Staff can remind residents of cues such as flowers on the bedroom door or pictures of grandchildren on a room sign that may help jog a resident's memory. Some residents, however, may not respond to any visual environmental cues, no matter how distinctive. Such people may not be able to make the connection between the cues and the fact that the cues indicate their rooms, or they might simply forget what they are seeking. In these cases, other strategies can be used. For example, if the next activity is a coffee klatch, then begin brewing coffee before the activity is scheduled to begin. This way, if a resident comes into the room or is directed there by staff, then he or she will be able to associate the aroma of the coffee with the activity at hand. Likewise, an exercise activity could be kicked off with the same song each time, the start of a baking program could be cued by baking a sheet of cookies in advance and letting the smell drift out of the activity area into the hallway. Who would not be drawn to the smell of freshly baked cookies?

Reality Orientation Versus Validation

It is important to help residents who have problems with orientation to believe that they have not completely lost themselves as a result of dementia. Many long-term care facilities use an approach known as *reality orientation* to help orient residents with dementia. This includes giving the correct information to a person who is confused about his or her current situation. An example of using reality orientation is telling a resident that her husband is deceased when she talks about him coming to visit. Whether a confused resident should be oriented to the present is debatable. In general, caution is advisable when using traditional reality orientation with residents with dementia.

Some residents with mild to moderate dementia may ask for orientation cues (e.g., "What day is today?", "Where are we?"); it is best to give them the accurate information. However, it is probably not effective to try to insist that they remember facts such as dates, seasons, and names. As cognitive impairment increases, reality orientation can sometimes do more harm than good. Telling residents with more severe dementia something other than what they believe to be true may only frighten or upset them.

> *Mrs. Rewick sometimes wanders the hallways saying that her husband is coming soon, but you know that he has been deceased for 5 years. Mrs. Rewick is disoriented to time and place (the current year and where she is). Saying to her, "Mrs. Rewick, you know your husband is dead, so he isn't coming today or ever," likely will be very upsetting to her because she has obviously forgotten this fact. She may even become so upset that she may try to leave the facility to find him.*

When staff encounter this situation, they should think carefully before deciding how to respond to Mrs. Rewick. It is possible that she may be talking about her husband because, deep down, she knows that he is dead, but she misses him and needs to feel close to him. It is also possible that she may not know that he is dead but is comforted by talking about him. An alternative response to reality orientation in these situations is to ask Mrs. Rewick about her husband. Talking about him may comfort her and may help her come to terms with his death. This type of approach, *validation*, which acknowledges Mrs. Rewick's feelings, often is preferable to traditional reality orientation, particularly in the later stages of a dementing illness.

> *Mrs. Epstein believes that she has young children that she must go home to feed, so she tries to leave the dementia unit every day around 5 P.M.*

Because Mrs. Epstein wants to go home and have dinner with her children, her wandering behavior can be redirected by getting her to help set the tables in the facility's dining room with napkins and place mats. In this way, she can still participate in preparing for dinner and still feel busy doing a chore that would be typical for her at that time of the day. "Renewing" or validating her role as a mother can be much more therapeutic for Mrs. Epstein than reminding her that she is living in a long-term care facility. (See Volume 4, Chapter 3 for an in-depth discussion of the importance of these roles in residents' lives.)

WHAT THE ENVIRONMENT CAN DO

Wayfinding in an unfamiliar environment can be a taxing experience for people of all ages. Think about how frustrated you are when you are trying to find a room in a hotel and all of the corridors look exactly the same and the signage is poor and hard to read. Residents with dementia who do not see or understand the environment in the same way as do people whose cognitive abilities remain intact are likely to have even greater difficulties in such settings.

Residents with dementia vary in terms of what characteristics of the environment they can still perceive at different stages of dementia. For example, some residents with early-stage dementia may have no trouble locating the bathroom, whereas other residents may experience great difficulties. Multiple cueing, or providing the same information in different ways (e.g., directed to several different senses), provides better information to more residents than would a single orientation cue. For instance, some residents are able to follow a sign indicating the direction to the toilet, others recognize a brightly colored canopy over the door, and still others need to be led by someone.

Experts are continually reevaluating strategies and types of cues. For example, several years ago it was thought that colored lines on the floor or wall could be an effective cue. However, this strategy may be difficult for many residents. It may be hard for them to see the line or to know which line to follow when there are several different lines. They may choose the color that they are most attracted to or can see best, which may take them to the dining room instead of the bathroom or vice versa. Residents also may forget that they are supposed to follow the line because this is not a cue that they would have used earlier in their lives.

This section discusses a number of general issues in navigating in a long-term care environment, including spatial adjacencies, color, and signage. The discussion is followed by an exploration of ways to make specific rooms easier to locate for residents with dementia.

Spatial Adjacencies

One important environmental issue is spatial adjacencies (how things are located in relationship to one another in a building) and how well the floor plan of the facility addresses the known problems of residents with dementia. Facilities often are restricted by the existing floor plan and cannot afford to build new units or even remodel existing ones significantly. However, some steps can be taken to make the existing environment more user-friendly for residents with dementia. Therefore, it is important to understand the strengths and drawbacks of different layouts in helping residents with dementia with orientation and wayfinding.

Double-Loaded Corridors

Most long-term care facilities have double-loaded corridors in which rooms are located on both sides of the hall (Figure 2.1). These corridors often stretch 50 feet or longer. Generally, long hallways are hard for people with dementia to navigate. When the doors on both sides of the hallway look similar, residents may have trouble locating their bedrooms or become disoriented easily. Impaired vision makes these problems worse because residents may not be able to find their destination when they cannot readily see it. Furthermore, residents with dementia may forget what they are seeking (e.g., dining room to eat dinner). These orientation problems can make residents both tired and frustrated. Some residents may simply give up looking for the location where an event is happening and miss out on the fun. Other residents may become agitated or even have catastrophic reactions.

A variety of steps can be taken to reduce the impact of double-loaded corridors on residents with dementia (see also Figure 2.2):

- Make important doorways more distinctive to attract the attention of residents with dementia (e.g., a three-dimensional canopy placed over the bathroom door that can be seen from down the hall).
- Provide plenty of unique landmarks, personalized cues, or both throughout the space. For instance, staff can remind Mrs. Carlson that her room is next to the quilt hanging on the wall. Check with the local fire marshal first to make sure that fire codes allow placement of items in the hallway. Items hung on the wall should not extend more

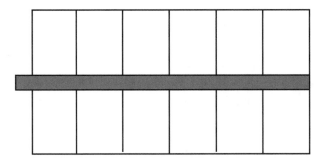

Figure 2.1.   Floor plan of a facility with double-loaded corridors.

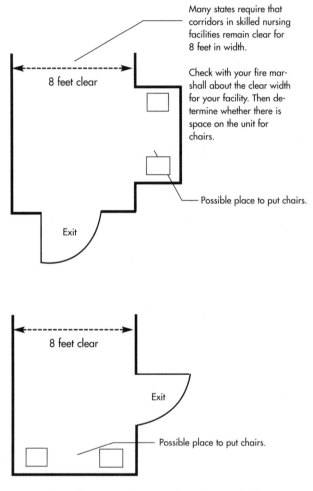

Many states require that corridors in skilled nursing facilities remain clear for 8 feet in width.

Check with your fire marshall about the clear width for your facility. Then determine whether there is space on the unit for chairs.

8 feet clear

Possible place to put chairs.

Exit

8 feet clear

Exit

Possible place to put chairs.

Figure 2.2.   Potential furniture locations in hallways.

than 4 inches into the hall to meet Americans with Disabilities Act of 1990 (ADA; PL 101-336, 42 U.S.C. §§ 12101 *et seq.*) standards.

- Create small seating areas along the hallways, if space permits, so that residents can stop and rest on the way to their destinations.
- Place interesting objects in the hallways (e.g., textured art) that residents can stop and touch; this may reduce their frustration about feeling lost in these areas.
- Treat each hallway differently. Use different colors, types of art, furniture, lighting fixtures—anything to make each hallway distinctive.

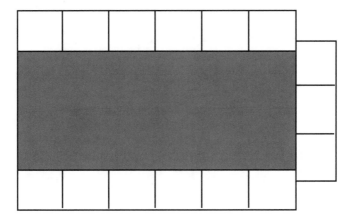

Figure 2.3.   Pavilion floor plan.

The stronger the contrast among hallways, the more effective these differences will be in serving as orientation cues.

Alternative Floor Plans

Because of the many challenges that are associated with double-loaded corridors, two alternative types of floor plans are described here. Facilities should consider the benefits of these plan types when planning renovations or new construction.

Pavilion Plan

The pavilion floor plan features a widened hallway that creates a large central open space with all bedrooms surrounding the central area (Figure 2.3). When residents walk out of their bedrooms, they immediately see the social spaces. The dining area may be centrally located and it may be set off by a low railing and a change in floor color. If there is a nursing station, it gives views of the whole space to enable staff to easily see how residents are doing. Orientation may be improved for residents with dementia because views of social spaces are more easily obtained from the residents' bedrooms.

It is possible to create a pseudo-pavilion plan in a facility that has a racetrack plan (see Figure 2.4). The racetrack plan is a variation of a double-loaded corridor in which all staff service spaces are located in the center of the building, around which runs a hallway that connects all of the residents' rooms. Racetrack plans frequently cause the same disorientation problems as double-loaded corridors. It may be possible to create pavilionlike areas by carving out social spaces in the service area. This can occur at the ends or in

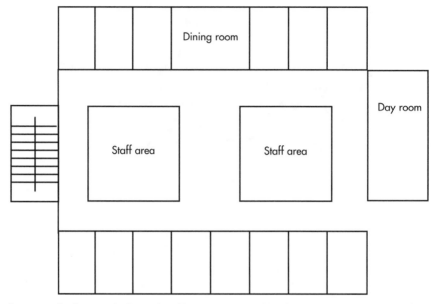

Before—Standard racetrack plan with staff spaces in the middle. ↑

After—Racetrack plan converted to a pavilion plan, which has better orientation and space for small groups. ↓

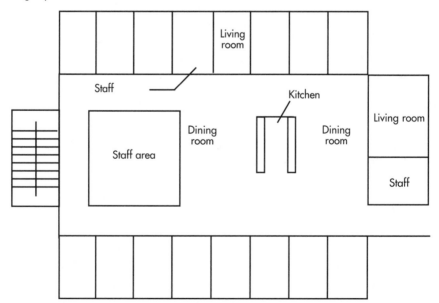

Figure 2.4.   Scheme for conversion from racetrack plan to pavilion plan.

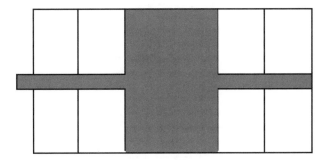

Figure 2.5.   Cluster floor plan.

the middle of the building. Not only will this floor plan variation assist residents with orientation but it may also help them concentrate on activities by dividing the common areas into smaller rooms.

Cluster Plan

Another type of floor plan clusters bedrooms around a central living area (Figure 2.5). This plan differs from a pavilion plan in that some bedrooms may be located along a hall; therefore, not all of the bedrooms on the unit open directly onto the living/activity rooms. Cluster plans are often used to break down the scale of large facilities into smaller households of 8–14 residents. Each cluster may have its own identity (e.g., color/theme/decorating scheme). The clustering of rooms around central living spaces is a pattern that is more residential than the traditional long-term care facility design, which features long hallways. Some clusters even have small dining rooms to provide family-style dining. It is easier in such a living arrangement to differentiate public areas (living and dining rooms) from private areas (bedrooms and bathrooms). The smaller scale of clusters helps to define a comfortable group size for social interaction and organized activities. Numerous guides that address the creation of effective settings for activity programming have shown that small-group activities are less overwhelming and more therapeutic for people with dementia (Brawley, 1997; Calkins, 1988; Cohen & Weisman, 1991).

If your facility has long double-loaded corridors with day rooms at the ends of the corridors, then it may be possible to convert this floor plan into a cluster design without undertaking major reconstruction (see Figure 2.6). The day room can be converted into a double or single bedroom, depending on its size, and either one or two bedrooms in the middle of the hall can be converted into a living room. Where building and life safety codes permit,

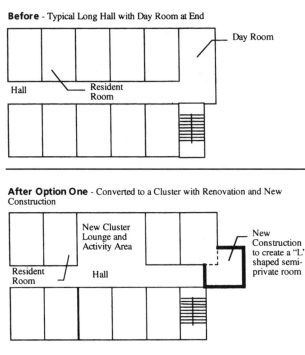

Before - Typical Long Hall with Day Room at End

Day Room

Hall

Resident Room

After Option One - Converted to a Cluster with Renovation and New Construction

New Cluster Lounge and Activity Area

Resident Room

Hall

New Construction to create a "L" shaped semi-private room

After - Option Two - Converted to a Cluster with Renovation Only

New Cluster Lounge

Resident Room

Hall

Figure 2.6. Scheme for conversion from typical double-loaded corridor plan to cluster plan.

the hallway wall could be removed and the living room area opened to the corridor. Where they do not, large interior windows and distinctive door treatments can be used. For this cluster living room to become an effective orientation cue, it needs to be used. Consider holding some "cluster-only" activities in this room or serving breakfast for late risers at a table in the cluster living room.

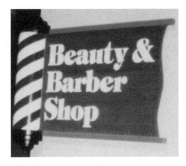

Figure 2.7. Example of a directional sign that is useful in assisting residents in wayfinding.

Cueing

Providing multiple orientation cues in the areas where residents with dementia live can increase their functional abilities significantly. Such cues may include

- Actual sight of the desired place and path to it
- Landmarks (furniture, color schemes, plants, artwork)
- Directional signs (see Figure 2.7)
- Sensory cues (e.g., smell of coffee brewing, sound of music playing)

Cues should be distinctive, varied, and bold because people with dementia often do not pick up on subtle cues (Brawley, 1997). For example, landmarks should be memorable objects in the environment, such as a bright, colorful quilt hanging in a hallway or a large fish tank in one corner. Staff can remind residents that these unique physical features can assist them in wayfinding. The overall goal is to make the environment user-friendly for residents so that staff do not need to act as guides repeatedly. (See "Where to Find Products" at the end of this chapter for sources of art that can be used as landmarks.)

Color

Color can be used to manage wayfinding problems in all areas of a unit. However, several issues must be considered when relying on color as an orientation cue. First, there is some controversy among designers regarding what colors are suitable for and easily perceived by residents with dementia. Second, color has no intrinsic meaning in everyday life, so a resident cannot always be expected to know that, for example, his or her room is on the blue hall. Third, some residents may be colorblind. Finally, people often are drawn to colors they prefer; therefore, it may be difficult to provide the right color for every resident on the unit. Carpman (1991) proposed the following useful tips when designing color-coding schemes:

- Keep it simple for wayfinding purposes.
- Use the same colors consistently. They should always have the same meaning and not be used in some places for meaning and in others just for decoration.
- Limit color coding to a few specific routes (e.g., path to the dining room).
- Use strongly contrasting colors so that older adults can see and differentiate easily between the colors. Subtle differences rarely will be noticed.

In general, color is used best when it is linked to the thematic concept of the design (e.g., blue for a wing with a boating theme). Also, color should be used in conjunction with other cueing schemes, such as a garden theme hallway that is painted green and decorated with floral patterns and lots of green plants. Staff also need to use these cues consistently when reminding residents where rooms are located.

Although color can be important for orientation and wayfinding, it also can help residents with low vision to understand the environment better. For example, using contrasting colors on the edges of furniture, on grab bars, and in hallways helps simplify the visual environment. This makes it easier for residents with low vision to concentrate on where they are going. This is particularly important when these residents also have dementia, and may have trouble focusing on multiple tasks at the same time. (See Volume 1, Chapter 2 for further ideas regarding the use of color contrast when designing safe environments.)

Signage

The notion that simply adding signs in the hallways will solve the problem of residents getting lost is a myth. In fact, having too many signs can be even more confusing, especially for residents with dementia. They often have trouble concentrating when there is too much information to process. Many design features also can make signs hard for older people to read. These features include small type, insufficient color contrast, confusing graphics, and poor sign placement in relation to lighting (Figure 2.8A).

When a facility is installing or replacing signs, they should be

- Large and easy to see

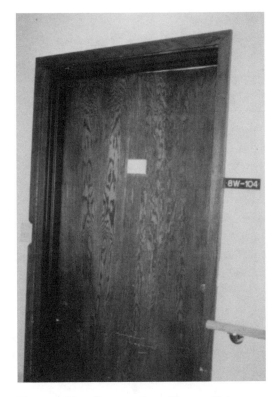

Figure 2.8A. Signage that will not aid in wayfinding. This sign has small letters and poor contrast and may be hard for residents to notice or read.

- Well placed
- Designed with realistic graphics
- Marked by good color contrast

A good combination for signs that are directed at residents includes dark lettering that is 2–3 inches high with dark graphics on a light background (Carpman, Grant, & Simmons, 1985). Graphics should be realistic rather than abstract (e.g., silverware for a dining room sign). Signs can be made of paper using different graphics at first to find out what works best before purchasing expensive printed signs (see "Where to Find Products" for sources of signage).

Signs should be placed where residents are most likely to see them. Many older adults will miss signs that are located on the upper sections of doors because they lack the range of head motion that younger people have.

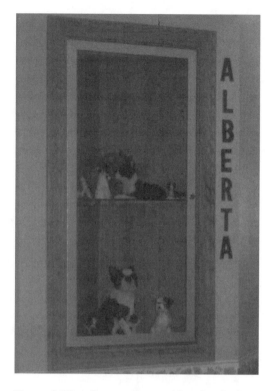

Figure 2.8B.   Signage as an aid to wayfinding.
This sign has large lettering and a shadow box
and includes cueing for the resident.

Another problem is that older adults may be stooped over from, for example, osteoporosis, and look downward when they walk. These residents likely will never see signs hung at ADA–approved height. You can supplement regulation signs by placing additional signs for these residents on the lower 24 inches of the wall or directly on the floor (Figure 2.8B).

Large signs should be used where they are necessary, expected, and needed. For example, it may not be necessary to label every lounge on the unit if each has a distinctive decor and location. Similarly, small dining rooms only for residents who live on the cluster are more in keeping with a home and are not normally labeled. Destinations such as the barber/beauty shop, the main dining room, the common bathroom, and activity rooms should be labeled. These are spaces that most people typically use signs to locate. Some residents may need reinforcement of signs with familiar cues (e.g., a red and white barber's pole for the men's barbershop).

Reducing Unnecessary Choices

Reducing the number of areas that residents have in view may enable them to more successfully locate the spaces they should use. If there are areas on the unit that the facility does not want residents to enter, then it may be advantageous to reduce the visual impact of the doorways to these areas. This can be accomplished by continuing the paint color or wall treatment that surrounds the opening across the door frame and the door.

Rooms

Locating Bedrooms

One of the major issues for people with dementia living in long-term care facilities is being able to locate their own bedrooms. The ability to independently locate one's room increases self-sufficiency and self-esteem. Yet residents with dementia often have trouble finding their bedrooms and distinguishing the correct bedroom from those of other residents. Wandering into others' bedrooms can increase anxiety and agitation and may lead to "borrowing" objects from the unfamiliar room. For these reasons, it is important to have good signage and other cueing systems in place to help residents locate their rooms. Ultimately, the placement of cues should be determined by the particular visual patterns and cognitive abilities of individual residents. Some residents may look only at the floor when they walk and therefore may not see signs or objects on the walls. Whatever is necessary to create a visually distinctive bedroom door and entry for each resident should be done.

First, good lighting enables residents to see bedroom signs, display cases, or other objects around the door that serve as personal cues for identifying their bedrooms. (See Volume 1, Chapter 2 for recommendations about types of lighting.) If doorways are located in deep recesses or lighting is poor, then the facility may want to consider installing lights at each door. Use frosted bulbs and lenses so that these lights do not create glare in the direct line of sight.

The second task is to determine the best signage and cueing system for making rooms distinctive for residents. A number of options are available. These include using signs, display shelves, display cabinets, and shadow boxes and creating distinctive bedroom interiors.

Signs
Signs should be placed on the middle or lower section of the bedroom door where residents are most likely to see them. For a resident who uses a wheel-

chair, signs should be no higher than 40–44 inches above the floor. Signs should be large and simple and have good visual contrast with the bedroom door. Dark lettering should be used on a light background, and letters should be at least 1 inch tall. Use residents' names as well as room numbers, and make sure that signs are securely attached to the door. Signs are available that incorporate a picture holder for resident photos. Facilities that are replacing their signs may want to consider this option. Alternatively, picture holders can be added to hallway walls by hanging inexpensive frames for standard-size pictures. Family members can then personalize these frames.

Display Options

Some facilities have installed small cabinets with shelves to give residents an opportunity to display some personal objects outside their bedroom entrances. Display cases reduce the institutional image of facility hallways. In addition, they can serve as orientation cues for residents with dementia. Display cases were first used at the Corinne Dolan Alzheimer Center in Chardon, Ohio, to encourage residents to find their rooms. These cases, which were adjacent to the bedroom door, were large and contained several glass shelves. Research has shown that the objects in these cases, if chosen carefully, can assist residents in finding their own rooms. Furthermore, the more significant the objects or the stronger residents' memories of them, the better these objects assisted residents with locating their own doors (Namazi, Rosner, & Rechlin, 1991).

Display cases can take the form of shadow boxes, curio cabinets, shelves, or display cases. Shadow boxes are thin cabinets with glass fronts, sometimes with shelves (Figure 2.9) (see "Where to Find Products" for sources). Curio cabinets have multiple shelves and may be open-fronted or may have glass doors. Display cabinets can take multiple forms and are usually larger than shadow boxes or curio cabinets. Some of these display cases can be purchased at home furnishings' stores. Many standard cabinets can be adapted for this use. The facility may want to have some cabinets built for specific needs and applications.

The type of display device that can be incorporated into a facility's hallways depends on the facility's physical design and budget. The most limited environment is the double-loaded corridor with doors. In facilities with this floor plan, the lowest cost option is to ask each resident's family to bring a picture from the resident's home and hang it outside the door. Another option is a shadow box or curio cabinet that is attached directly to the wall and filled with items that a resident can identify with or recognize (Figure 2.10, Option

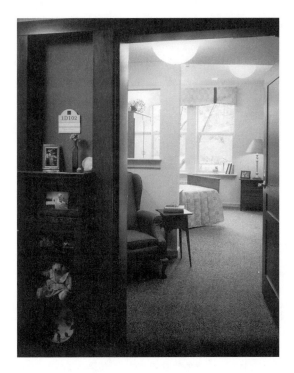

Figure 2.9.   A shadow box located outside a resident's room.

One). The cabinets should have glare-free glass so that objects inside them are easily visible. ADA requires that these cabinets not intrude more than 4 inches into the hallway. There is no reason that all of the cabinets must look the same. Consider purchasing a variety of styles so that the type of cabinet also helps residents distinguish their own doors.

A more expensive and more effective method is to use a deeper cabinet recessed into the wall (Figure 2.10, Option Two). Recessed cabinets are sometimes restricted by wall construction, building codes, and cost. If the facility was built with stud walls, then the best choice is recessed cabinets that will fit in the space between the studs (usually 16 inches apart). Before installing recessed cabinets, consult with an architect or contractor to determine what is possible and what is allowed by local building codes.

If the facility has doors that are recessed from the hall, then it may be possible to use this recessed area for personalization (see Figure 2.10, Options Three and Four). Recessed doorways may have room for a shelf, a shadow box, or a display cabinet that will not prevent residents from using

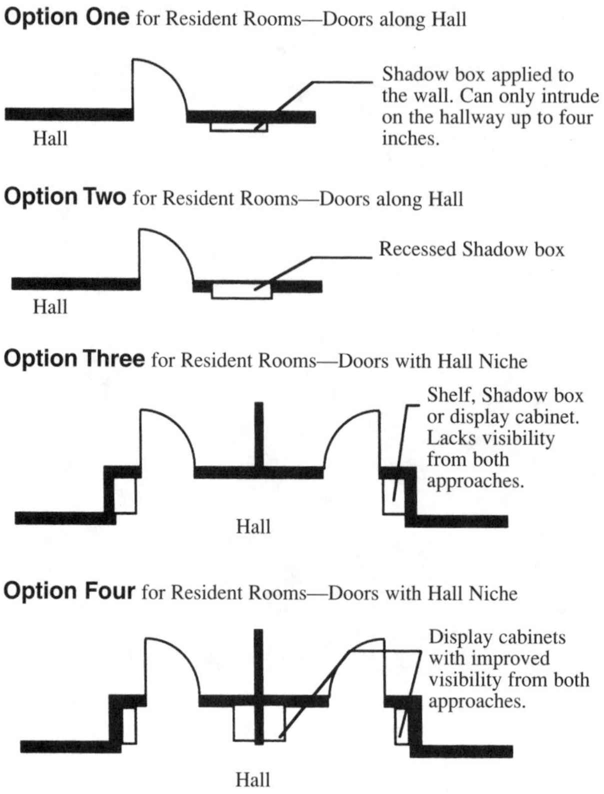

Option One for Resident Rooms—Doors along Hall

Hall

Shadow box applied to the wall. Can only intrude on the hallway up to four inches.

Option Two for Resident Rooms—Doors along Hall

Hall

Recessed Shadow box

Option Three for Resident Rooms—Doors with Hall Niche

Hall

Shelf, Shadow box or display cabinet. Lacks visibility from both approaches.

Option Four for Resident Rooms—Doors with Hall Niche

Hall

Display cabinets with improved visibility from both approaches.

Figure 2.10. Options for placement of display cabinets near residents' room doors.

the door. The simplest and least expensive option is to install a niche or alcove shelf. Residents and their families may enjoy selecting artwork or small objects to place on the shelf and in the alcove. However, if some residents on the unit rummage, then it may not be possible to use shelves. Instead, an enclosed display cabinet or curio cabinet can be installed, or, for facilities with sufficient funds and ample space, it may be possible to build customized cabinets. In the latter case, they should consider installing interior lights and using glass shelves to help residents to see the objects inside. Try to locate cabinets so that some items can be seen from both approaches coming down the hall.

Distinctive Bedroom Interiors
Residents are more likely to enter the correct room if the bedroom is painted in their favorite color or colors and decorated with favorite pieces of art and

personal objects from home. Some research has suggested that personally meaningful cues are up to 50% more effective than nonpersonal cues in assisting residents in finding their bedrooms (Namazi et al., 1991). This study found that residents understood personal cues such as a favorite chair better than symbolic or abstract cues such as pictures of favorite animals or a vacation spot.

A resident's bedroom should be visually pleasing and reflect his or her own sense of style. The facility may be able to offer several color choices for painting bedroom walls for residents in private rooms. Residents with dementia usually do best when they can choose from a range of three to five colors. Provide large sheets of colored paper among which residents can choose rather than small paint chips, which are harder to see. Sometimes residents with impaired communication skills may not be able to tell you which color they prefer. One way to judge their color preferences is to give them some different-colored objects (e.g., fabric swatches) and see which colors they pick up and handle most. You can also ask family members to tell you residents' lifelong color preferences or ask to see photos of their previous homes. It is likely that residents will prefer the same color schemes in which their homes were decorated. In general, it is better when adjacent resident bedrooms are painted different colors so that residents do not become confused. If the facility cannot afford the time and money to repaint the rooms, or if the majority of the rooms are semiprivate, then other options can be chosen for differentiating bedrooms. Bedspreads, blankets, privacy curtains, and window curtains usually can be changed easily and are available in a variety of colors and patterns. This may be a more familiar decorating scheme for residents whose house walls were always white and used color in their furniture fabrics.

Many residents respond to photographs of themselves. Some may respond to recent pictures, whereas others may respond only to pictures of themselves from an earlier time. Engagement, wedding, and birthday pictures are often good choices, and they can be provided by family members. When a resident responds to a picture, hang it on the room sign or to the side of the bedroom door in an easily visible location. Some residents may not recognize their pictures but might respond to a picture of their house or a favorite pet, or even an object such as a wreath from home. Ask families for input in selecting an appropriate object (e.g., if the person was a florist, hang a nosegay of dried flowers on the door). A resident also might respond to something that he or she made, such as a drawing from an art therapy session.

Locating Bathrooms

Being able to locate bathrooms is important for residents. It gives them the opportunity to be more independent and reduces accidents, which are un-

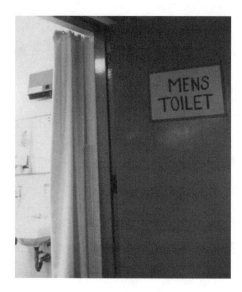

Figure 2.11A.   Signage for locating bathrooms. Depending on the facility's layout, it may be necessary to distinguish men's and women's bathrooms.

pleasant for residents and staff alike. Residents with dementia are more likely to remember to use toilets that are visible and easy for them to find. Whenever possible, bathrooms should be located both close to shared living areas (e.g., dining room) and in bedrooms. There should be a clear distinction made between the men's room and the women's room in common bathrooms located in shared living areas, or residents will enter the wrong room (Figure 2.11A). This is especially true if the two bathrooms are adjacent.

Staff should do whatever is necessary to make the bathroom more visually distinctive and draw the attention of residents. This may include painting the door a bright color, using a different treatment from all of the other doors, or placing eye-catching graphics/signs on the door and the floor (Figure 2.11B). Make sure that modifications are visually bold so that residents with low vision can see them more easily. For example, a three-dimensional canopy increases the visibility of the bathroom from down the hall. Canopies usually can be constructed from standard drapery and hardware. Staff should be creative in trying these suggestions as well as other physical orientation aids to help cue residents to the location of the bathroom. As residents become more demented, it is likely that staff will need to escort residents to the bathroom, but it is important to promote the residents' own functional abilities as long as possible.

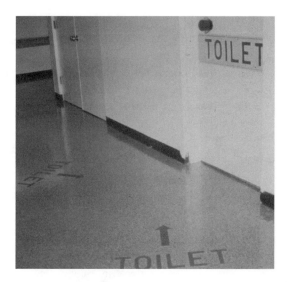

Figure 2.11B. Signage for locating bathrooms. Large graphics and multiple signs help draw residents' attention.

Once the resident is in the bathroom, the next issue is for him or her to be able to locate the toilet. There are a number of ways to make the toilet more visible, including replacing doors with curtains that can be pulled back, making the toilet seat a contrasting color from the tank and bowl, or installing a night light that draws attention to the toilet. (See Chapter 4 in this volume for a more extensive discussion of ways to minimize incontinence with environmental and behavioral interventions.)

Locating Dining Rooms

Mealtimes are one of the most consistent routines for residents in long-term care facilities, yet residents with dementia may have trouble locating the dining room. Providing cues that help these residents to find their way to the dining room will increase their feelings of competence. Signs with large bold lettering and simple graphics (e.g., a picture of a place setting) can help residents to find the dining room. Staff should try different things and see what works with their residents. Probably the most effective type of cue for the dining room is the aroma of food cooking. This does not mean the whole meal must be prepared on the unit. Brew a pot of coffee, use a bread maker, bake some rolls in a toaster oven, or consider cutting an onion in half and heating it in a toaster oven. All of the resulting aromas will tell residents it is mealtime and will help them to find their way to the dining room.

Residents can more easily recognize a dining room if it looks like a dining room rather than a multipurpose room. Dining rooms in people's homes frequently have a large hutch filled with china or dishes. Residents may be able to identify a dining room better if this piece of furniture is placed in it. If the dining room is also used as an activities room, try to change its appearance or provide special cues to indicate when it is mealtime. For example, place brightly colored place mats or tablecloths on the tables. Some residents may enjoy assisting in this activity. Use other sensory cues such as playing a certain piece of music before meals.

Locating Shared Living Spaces

To increase residents' quality of life, it is important to help them find places to socialize with others on the unit. Residents are less likely to socialize if they have trouble finding the shared living spaces on the unit. Staff and volunteers should make sure to invite residents to activity programs and give simple directions about how to get there, or go with the residents to make sure that they can find the way. It is important to use terminology with which the residents are likely to be familiar, such as "living room" instead of "day room." Decorate these rooms so their function is more obvious (e.g., have chairs arranged in small groups rather than lined up along the walls, which gives an institutional appearance).

The locations of the shared living areas in many facilities were designed to permit the staff to have direct visual access to these areas. Consequently, the living room or day room on many units is located next to a nurses' station. As a result, residents may congregate around the nursing area because it is a center of activity rather than using the designated living room. Staff should try to make this living room more attractive and homelike. If possible, the facility also should set up several smaller social areas in other locations on the unit and encourage residents to go to these areas. These smaller areas will generally be less overwhelming and more enjoyable for residents. Make each area visually distinctive—a sun porch with wicker rockers and plants or a library/den with magazines and books in bookcases (Figure 2.12).

There has long been debate about whether visual barriers between spaces are a good idea. Some argue that it is important to have direct visual access to shared areas, so that residents can see what is going on and decide whether to stop by and participate or watch. It is thought that direct visual access may facilitate wayfinding by increasing residents' orientation capacity (Lawton et al., 1984; Leibowitz et al., 1979). Others believe that direct visual access may distract residents with dementia and make it hard for them to concentrate on an activity. The facility should try to accommodate both patterns.

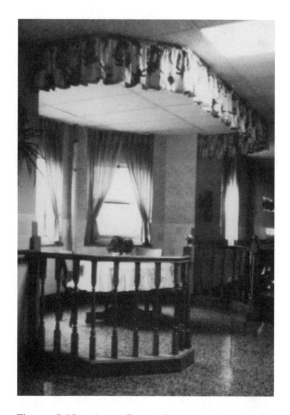

Figure 2.12. A small social area made visually distinctive with a railing, curtains, tablecloth, and canopy.

For residents who are easily distracted, try to hold small activities in rooms with the door shut. However, if all of the doors to activity rooms are solid, then the facility may want to consider installing doors with glass to provide residents with visual access to activities.

Locating Outdoor Spaces

Many residents with dementia still enjoy going outside to sit in the warm sunshine or enjoy the changing of the seasons. Being able to go outside can provide a rich sensory experience for these residents. Yet, too often, residents with dementia have limited access to the outdoors because of rules and restrictions or their inability to figure out how to get outside and return. The best solution is to have direct, unrestricted access to an enclosed courtyard. If residents are able to see the courtyard from common spaces, then it is more likely to be used by all. Staff also may feel more comfortable about letting residents go outside if staff can see easily into the courtyard.

Staff need to be creative in thinking of ways to encourage residents to find their way to these outside spaces. Make sure that courtyards for the residents can be seen easily from the unit (e.g., hang sheer curtains on the windows so that glare is minimized but there is still a good view to the outdoors with light coming in the window). Good visual access to the outdoors through windows also helps orient residents to both the time of day and the season. Transition areas from indoors to outdoors should be well lit and provide a place for older people to stop and rest while their eyes adjust to the change in light levels.

The ground surfaces should be as level as possible so that residents can enjoy nature rather than focusing on navigating along the path. Paths should be laid out so that they always return to the building if the facility has a large area with multiple paths for resident use. Provide a special landmark at critical junctions, such as a red resting bench (a red bench is unusual and may stand out).

Outdoor spaces can include different types of orientation cues that remind residents of being in their own backyards or sitting on the front porch. These cues include pleasant seating areas along the path, brightly colored beach umbrellas for providing shade, or seasonal plantings. White plastic tables produce glare and make it hard for residents to see when they are sitting at them. Covering these tables with a brightly colored vinyl tablecloth provides more contrast between the table surface and the ground and helps residents to see the tables more easily when they are on the path. Volumes 3 and 4 of this series provide more information on how to create therapeutic outdoor areas.

WHERE TO FIND PRODUCTS

Creating Landmarks with Artwork

Artline
W227 North 937 Westmound Drive
Waukesha, WI 53186
(800) 795-9596
www.artline.com
Interactive and memory-based artwork

DesignXpertise Studio
1700 Mary Street
Pittsburgh, PA 15203
(412) 431-5733
www.designxpertise.com
Memory quilts and memory boxes by artist Karen Scofield

3D Interactive Art by Mardel DeBuhr Sanzotta
84 Fruitland Avenue
Painesville, OH 44077
(216) 357-7122
Tactile artwork with some interactive items

Signage

EMED Co., Inc.
Post Office Box 369
Buffalo, NY 14240-0369
(800) 442-3633
www.emedco.com
A variety of standard facility signs and custom signs

Graphics Systems Inc.
313 Ida
Wichita, KS 67211
(316) 267-4171
www.gsi-graphics.com

Kaltech Industries Group, Inc.
Kaltech Architectural Signage
123 West 19th Street
New York, NY 10011
(800) 435-TECH
www.kaltech.com/framset.htm
Modular sign systems that can be customized

Scott Sign Systems, Inc.
Post Office Box 1047
Tallevast, FL 34270-1047
(800) 237-9447
www.scottsigns.com

Shadow Boxes

> **Exposures, Inc.**
> Post Office Box 3615
> Oshkosh, WI 54903-3615
> (800) 222-4947
> *www.exposuresonline.com*
> A catalog of items for the storage and display of photographs and mementos

◆ ◆ ◆

A summary sheet follows, which condenses the chapter text into a quick overview. The authors have also provided an area for you to make your own notes about your own staff and facility. Managerial staff may wish to use the summary sheets as handouts to accompany direct care staff training, or to post them by the time clock or nurses' station or include them in staff's pay envelopes.

ORIENTATION SUMMARY SHEET

1. Orientation refers to knowing and understanding the world.
2. A person is oriented to people if he or she can identify him- or herself and can recognize other people, especially significant others.
3. Orientation to time refers to year, month, or season, and day and/or date.
4. Orientation to place includes home address, where one is currently, or how to find one's bedroom.
5. Wayfinding is using environmental information to reach a desired destination.
6. Agnosia, difficulty in telling things apart, often occurs with dementia. If the trouble is visual, then the person may not recognize a spouse, children, or home.
7. Visuospatial problems (judging where objects begin and end) and difficulty in making new mental maps also interfere with wayfinding.
8. Disorientation to time can make it difficult for people with dementia to wait.
9. Some people with dementia ask for assistance with orientation. Others can be quite upset or frightened by reality orientation.

What Staff Can Do

1. Increase environmental sensory cues (smells, sounds) to help disoriented residents find/relate to events when they become socially withdrawn.
2. Remind residents of the special environmental cues that identify their hall or room.

What the Environment Can Do

1. Make important doorways distinctive and three-dimensional when possible.
2. Provide unique landmarks and personal cues.
3. Create rest areas where possible in long hallways or along paths to activity areas.
4. Provide interesting objects and tactile opportunities.
5. Reduce the chance of residents' getting lost by offering or including actual sight of a destination: landmarks such as furniture and clearly marked, well-placed directional signs, and sensory information (e.g., coffee brewing, music playing).
6. Help to identify resident rooms by using appropriate signs, adequate lighting, personal photos/objects on doors/in frames/display cases, distinctive interiors, and personal furnishings or objects.
7. Enable residents to find toilets (critical for self-respect and staff's efficiency) by making them easy to spot: paint doors bright colors, use canopies or interesting signs, make toilet seats contrast with other fixtures and walls, and leave lights on or use night-lights.

8. Create shared spaces and programs so that residents are more likely to socialize. Small, intimate spaces are more comfortable for some residents.

9. Provide access to outdoor areas. Make doors easily visible, make walking surfaces smooth, make it easy for staff to see the area, provide comfortable seating and shade, and make sure that there are interesting things to see and do.

YOUR NOTES

3
Mobility

Most of us take mobility for granted. We seldom stop to consider what life would be like if we could not freely go where we wanted or do what we wished to do. Yet people with mobility problems often have difficulties performing basic activities such as walking, getting out of a bed or chair, using a toilet, or bathing. Such mobility problems not only threaten people's ability to perform their activities of daily living (ADLs) but also can have a deep psychological impact. It is frustrating not to be able to do what you want to do easily, or always to need to plan activities around whether various places will be accessible to you.

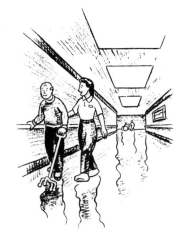

Many younger people only become aware of what mobility problems are like when they have accidents (e.g., breaking a leg) that temporarily cause them to experience these daily challenges. After a debilitating injury, they often learn how difficult it can be, for example, to get dressed, drive to work, or carry a cup of coffee while using crutches. Under these circumstances, even the relatively short distance from a handicapped-access parking space into a building can seem to last forever. Having these types of problems for just a few weeks can really make them appreciate their mobility. What would your life be like if you suddenly developed a disability and always had to use crutches? Thinking about the many ways in which this would affect your daily routine will help you to be more sensitive to residents who must live with permanent mobility problems.

MOBILITY IN OLDER PEOPLE

In older adults, mobility problems may develop gradually (e.g., increased unsteadiness when walking) or occur suddenly (e.g., a hip fracture). Mobility problems can have a great impact on numerous areas of an older person's life, including functional abilities, psychological well-being, and personal autonomy. It can be a serious problem for an older person living alone when he or she can no longer easily climb the stairs to reach the bedroom on the second floor or descend the stairs to the basement to do laundry. No longer being able to do the necessary activities for running the household can be depressing for an older person. Acknowledging new limitations and realizing that these may be permanent changes can be difficult.

Many older people who still live in the community also worry about whether such mobility problems will affect their ability to live independently. As mobility problems worsen, psychological conditions, including lethargy, passivity, social withdrawal, and depression, occur commonly. Some older adults may cease to go out at all because it is too difficult for them to get around or because they fear falling. This can lead to isolation, loneliness, and a diminished quality of life.

Facing the reality of needing to live in a long-term care facility is hard for many older adults. They often fear that they will not be able to maintain their own lifestyles after they move to a more physically supportive setting. Although some actually may feel safer after moving into a facility, residents with mobility problems still face numerous psychological and physiological issues.

Psychological Issues

Like younger people, many older adults greatly value their independence and do not like to have to rely on others. Consequently, the self-image and self-confidence of residents with mobility problems often are affected negatively. They may feel vulnerable, helpless, angry, frustrated, or bitter about their losses. It can be quite difficult for them to accept that they may need more time, more help, and possibly specialized equipment just to be able to get around in their environment. It can be intensely frustrating for older people when they can no longer easily do things that they have been used to doing for many years.

Residents with mobility problems often can continue to safely do many of the activities that they enjoy. Maintaining these lifelong patterns can be psychologically beneficial and can help them to maintain their self-esteem. For example, a serious bowler can safely become a wheelchair bowler; a lifelong gardener can grow plants in raised beds. Participating in favorite activities often helps residents focus on their skills and expertise rather than on their losses. Whereas some residents may not want to make these compromises, others welcome the opportunity to remain active. This is a highly personal decision that each resident needs to make for him- or herself.

Physiological Issues

Mobility generally involves several physical systems operating together: musculoskeletal, neurological, cardiovascular, and sensory. A number of age-related problems pertaining to each of these systems can affect mobility negatively. An excellent practical resource that describes these problems in detail is *Falls in Older Persons: Prevention & Management* (Tideiksaar, 1998). His discussion of these issues is summarized in this section.

Age-related musculoskeletal changes can affect overall mobility levels. Muscle mass decreases with advancing age. Older people who become less physically active are more likely to have muscle atrophy and weakness from disuse. When an older person experiences prolonged bed rest or immobility, such weakness is more likely to occur. Similarly, when bones do not bear weight over time, a process of bone deterioration known as osteoporosis can take place. This condition is very serious because it increases the risk of fractures. It affects women more than men, but it also is a serious concern for older men.

Although many people do not think of neurological problems as being related to mobility, the two issues can be integrally linked. For example, problems with balance and falling often have a neurological component. In some cases, mobility problems are actually the first symptoms that alert physicians that a neurological problem also may exist.

Failure to maintain an adequate blood supply to the brain can worsen mobility problems. Hypertension, hypotension, and other related disorders can produce a sensation of light-headedness affecting both balance and mobility when older people stand up. Older people with cardiovascular problems also tend to lower their overall mobility levels because they become easily fatigued. Ultimately, this physical deconditioning can negatively affect their mobility.

Mobility problems often are magnified by sensory impairments. Because sensory cues help us to interpret the physical environment, these losses may result in instability, confusion, and disorientation. An older person's poor vision may interfere with walking and transferring safely. Impaired hearing and diminished tactile sense also can affect mobility negatively. All of these conditions can make residents prone to falling.

The connection between poor balance and high rates of falling in older people is well documented. The goal of balance is to position the body's center of gravity over its base of support. Maintaining balance is dependent on a variety of central nervous system mechanisms. The roles of the central nervous system are to process sensory information and to initiate an appropriate response that enables the person to retain balance and stay upright.

Research studies have shown that older people experience more unsteadiness and problems with balance than younger people, even when standing still (Tideiksaar, 1998). Cognitive impairments may further worsen difficulties. The need to pay attention to more than one thing at a time may interfere with an older person's posture and balance.

Older people also often experience significant changes in their gait. Muscle weakness, pain, and fatigue can contribute to changes in gait. Psychological factors, such as an increased fear of falling, also can cause older adults to alter their gait. Some problems that are observed frequently in older people with gait disorders include short, shuffling steps and staggering, swaying, or lurching when walking. Numerous aspects of gait can be evaluated, including

- Step length
- Step height
- Step width
- Continuity
- Symmetry
- Ability to turn around
- Ability to pick up speed

Foot pain also may cause older people to change their gait, resulting in unsteadiness and lack of balance. Foot conditions such as corns, calluses, bunions, and toe and nail deformities can cause pain and contribute to mobility problems. Poorly fitting shoes also may cause foot pain. Most foot conditions are treatable, and require evaluation by appropriate medical personnel.

Older people often take multiple medications, and these combinations of drugs can cause mobility problems. The use of psychotropic medications such as sedatives and antidepressants, which are linked to an increased risk of falling, should be carefully monitored in older adults. Older people also more frequently experience adverse reactions to these medications, even at reduced dosages. Several other classes of medications, including diuretics and antihypertensives, that are widely prescribed for older people may increase their risk of falling. These drugs cause older adults to need to use the toilet both more frequently and urgently, resulting in more falls in bathrooms.

Falls

Falls are a major source of disability in older adults. A substantial amount of epidemiological research since the mid-1980s has shown that the frequency of falls increases with advancing age. Older people may fall as a result of age-related physiological changes or because of external factors such as hazardous environmental conditions or faulty mobility aids and devices. In many cases, falls result from a combination of physiological and environmental factors (Tideiksaar, 1998). Most older people fall while doing common everyday activities such as walking; transferring from chairs, beds, and toilets; performing ADLs (e.g., bathing); or bending over to reach things. Certain older people are more vulnerable to these problems. For example, older people with mobility impairments and reduced functional abilities have higher risks of falling (Morse, Tylko, & Dixon, 1987).

Research has shown that residents are most likely to fall shortly after moving into a long-term care facility. One study showed that up to one third of resident falls occurred within the first 45 days of admission (Gray-Micelli, Waxman, Cavalieri, & Lage, 1994). Rates of falling are affected by a number of situational factors, including the length of stay in the long-term care facility, familiarity with the layout of the environment, time of day, and staff-to-resident ratio (Tideiksaar, 1998). Falls can have lasting physical and psychological consequences for residents. Older people recover more slowly from these injuries and many experience difficulties regaining prior levels of physical function. Some of the more common physical injuries from falling include hip fractures, lower forearm or wrist fractures, and head trauma. More than 250,000 hip fractures occur each year in older Americans (Burns et al., 1997). Tideiksaar (1998) stated that factors influencing the likelihood of a fracture include

- The way the person falls
- The height of the fall
- Use of protective reflexes (e.g., extending arms)
- The weight of the individual
- The type of floor surface (e.g., linoleum versus carpet)

Individual characteristics can also influence the outcomes of falls. These include the number of previous falls, bone density, and degree of neuromuscular and cognitive deficits.

One of the best preventive strategies for reducing the number of falls is to maintain or improve residents' overall physical conditioning. Numerous studies have shown that exercise can be beneficial for older adults, including those with mobility problems. Some of these benefits include improved lung capacity and oxygenation; increased stamina and endurance; improved cardiac output, muscle tone, digestion, and elimination; and decreased bone loss, glucose intolerance risk, hypertension, depression, and stress (Payten & Porter, 1994). Exercises that emphasize muscular strength, joint flexibility, and sensory interaction are especially helpful for residents who suffer from gait and balance problems. Weight-bearing exercises are beneficial in reducing the rate of bone loss and lowering the risk of fractures. Exercise can help in preventing osteoporosis, which is linked to many fractures of the hip, spine, and extremities in older adults. A moderate weight-bearing exercise program assists in maintaining and increasing bone mass. The most common weight-bearing activity is walking, but there are many other alternatives for residents who experience difficulties in walking but want to exercise.

Another positive benefit of exercise in older adults is muscle strengthening. Research has shown that older people retain their ability to increase muscle strength through exercise. There is a significant relationship between strength training and increased lower extremity muscle strength. Even light resistance and stretching exercises of the legs can improve lower extremity flexibility and strength. Regular low-intensity exercise programs (including seated ones) can strengthen quadriceps muscles, improve joint flexibility, and play a role in increasing functional capacity (Tideiksaar, 1998). Such training can also improve gait and balance. The positive effects of muscle strengthening can benefit frail people as well as healthy ones.

MOBILITY IN OLDER PEOPLE WITH DEMENTIA

People with dementia are at a higher risk than other older adults for certain mobility problems. For example, research indicates that there is a higher incidence of falls among residents with dementia than among those without dementia (Morse et al., 1987). Because of their cognitive difficulties, these residents may forget to take necessary precautions such as rising slowly from a seated position or asking for assistance. Even in the early stage, residents with dementia may experience balance and gait disturbances. Learning how to use mobility aids or other assistive devices also can be especially challenging for these residents.

Apraxia

Residents with dementia frequently suffer from *apraxia,* a neurological condition that affects motor-planning skills. They may have difficulties remembering how to perform routine motor tasks such as transferring from beds, chairs, and toilets and walking. Because their brains do not process nerve impulses correctly, these residents may experience mobility problems even when their levels of strength and sensation are sufficient for these tasks. Common symptoms of apraxia are walking in place instead of moving forward or the feet appearing to be stuck to the floor. In the early stage of the dementing illness these changes may be perceived as clumsiness, but later apraxia can cause a severe lack of coordination and balance.

Risk of Falling in Residents with Dementia

When residents with dementia also have mobility problems, their risk of falling is greatly increased. These residents often have trouble focusing on multiple steps of a task at the same time. For instance, toileting involves a series of steps requiring both mobility and cognition: getting up from a chair or bed, going to the bathroom, adjusting clothing, transferring to and from the toilet, readjusting clothing, and exiting the bathroom. (A full discussion of toileting problems is provided in Chapter 4.) It may be difficult for residents with dementia to concentrate on each of these steps without losing their balance. "What the Environment Can Do" examines ways to make bathrooms safer.

Restraints

Long-term care facilities traditionally have used restraints to minimize residents' risks of falling as their dementia progressed. In many instances the use of restraints conflicts with a resident's right to autonomy and dignity. Since the mid-1980s, attitudes toward restraint use have changed greatly, spurred in large part by the mandates of the Omnibus Budget Reconciliation Act (OBRA) of 1987. This act provided federal guidelines on the use of restraints in nursing facilities. Before the passage of OBRA, studies showed that restraint usage ranged between 19% and 85% in U.S. nursing facilities (Dube & Mitchell, 1986). Restraints often were used for other than therapeutic reasons (e.g., the convenience of the staff). Furthermore, residents with greater cognitive impairments were more likely to be restrained frequently. Now it is widely recognized that using restraints is rarely the best solution, and restraint-free environments are promoted.

There are both mechanical and chemical restraints. Mechanical restraints constrain a person's ability to function or move freely. These include wheelchair restraints, belts, vests or chest jackets, mitts, side rails, and geriatric chairs with fixed tray tables. Chemical restraints include a variety of psychotropic medications. Psychotropic medications do have therapeutic uses in some older residents (e.g., treating depression), but they must be used correctly and not abused. Some older people may have adverse reactions to psychotropic medications. For example, if the dosage level is not appropriate, they may experience "reversible confusion." This is a form of excess disability because it occurs as a result of restraint use, not disease.

Being forced to wear mechanical restraint devices often makes residents feel like prisoners or children. To a resident with dementia, physical restraints may look like instruments of punishment. Residents have lived long lives filled with all kinds of experiences that shape their perceptions. If a resident was physically abused in his or her younger years, then he or she may have a catastrophic reaction if even shown a restraint. To understand how residents feel when they are restrained, staff should try spending 2 hours in a restraint after a meal to see what the experience is actually like. The impact of this experience is likely to be more powerful than any other form of training in restraint reduction.

Although the goal of restraint use may be to enhance residents' safety, both the physical and psychological harm of using restraints is often not worth it. The consequences of restraint use for residents with dementia are particularly serious because these residents often have impaired communication skills. Therefore, they may not be able to indicate when restraints cause them either physical or psychological pain. Studies have shown that people in restraints may quickly develop problems relating to physical immobility, including pressure sores, incontinence, muscle atrophy, skin problems, general deconditioning, decreased circulation, and, in the worst case, unintentional death by strangulation (Braun & Lipson, 1993).

Because a restrained person has less possibility for environmental stimulation, cognitive function may be reduced along with physical condition (Wykle, 1993). Using restraints can also trigger negative emotional responses ranging from fear and panic to humiliation and social withdrawal. Restraints may promote agitated behavior and catastrophic reactions in residents. These adverse psychological consequences are also bad for residents' physical health (Braun & Lipson, 1993). Residents who are restrained are also more likely to suffer from self-image problems. It is degrading for anyone to be restrained. Residents who are restrained frequently may exhibit negative behaviors more often, including

- An increased desire to exit
- Combative behavior
- Confusion
- Paranoia
- Higher levels of agitation

Finally, even people with dementia can pick up social cues regarding how others perceive them. Being restrained gives others the impression that these residents are dangerous, unpredictable, and to be avoided. In fact, restrained residents may be so deeply embarrassed that they withdraw from socializing completely. For all of these reasons, other strategies besides restraint use that are more therapeutic for residents should be considered.

Exercise and rehabilitation are two more therapeutic strategies for enhancing the safety of these residents. Some readers may dismiss these options as being either too expensive or inappropriate for these residents. However, improving the overall physical functioning of residents with dementia is key both for maintaining their current levels of mobility and reducing the overall amount of staff assistance that they need (e.g., continuing at the level of a one-person transfer versus requiring a two-person transfer). The following paragraphs summarize some of the benefits of each of these approaches.

Exercise

For residents with dementia and mobility problems, exercise can serve both as a form of physical conditioning and as an enjoyable social event. Beyond the improvement of general health and well-being, exercise can help improve socialization, attention span, sleep patterns, and wandering, and minimizes depression and aggression. Exercise also can provide opportunities for self-expression. Exercise programs can add structure and routine, which are so important for residents with dementia.

Research has shown that most residents with dementia do better in smaller exercise programs in which people with similar levels of cognitive impairment are grouped together. Smaller exercise groups are beneficial in that there is more individual attention, less sensory overload, and more visual recognition of consistent staff. Residents with dementia may do better when there are two or three smaller/shorter exercise programs offered instead of a longer activity. For example, they may benefit more from two 15-minute programs as opposed to one 30-minute program.

The hearing, visual, and cognitive deficits of these residents sometimes cause them to experience confusion and anxiety in activity programs. If residents cannot hear the activity leader or the music, then they easily become distracted and agitated and may have trouble participating in the program. If the exercise program uses fairly loud music, then the noise level may be distracting and uncomfortable for residents who use hearing aids. Similarly, when residents cannot see the exercise leader, they may become confused or lose interest in the program. They may become embarrassed or upset when they have trouble following along. Therefore, to get the maximum benefit from these programs, it is important to consider the needs of each resident.

Rehabilitation

Many residents with dementia become less physically active, resulting in deconditioning and functional decline (Tappen et al., 1997). Reasons that residents with dementia in long-term care facilities may become increasingly physically inactive include pathological conditions, cognitive deficits, and depression. In too many facilities these residents simply are allowed to decline until they are so weak that there is little or no possibility for rehabilitation.

Traditionally, people with dementia have not been considered good candidates for rehabilitation, and their physical needs in this area often go unaddressed. Yet many residents with dementia could benefit significantly from rehabilitation and could continue performing ADLs longer if they participated in a therapeutic rehabilitation program. In general, it is less costly for a facility to promote residents' remaining functional abilities than to provide more skilled levels of care.

The needs of residents with dementia must be addressed when designing their rehabilitation programs. In terms of stamina and endurance, residents with dementia are not necessarily different from other residents of similar ages. Maintaining their concentration and coordination may require them to expend more effort than residents without dementia. Their rehabilitation sessions should be short and should emphasize the skills and functional abilities that are most important for them. These residents commonly have trouble doing multiple tasks simultaneously. For example, when they are concentrating on instructions, they may have trouble with the secondary task of maintaining balance. Simple step-by-step instructions make it easier for them to focus on the task at hand. Rehabilitation also may be easier if they are shown rather than told what to do, especially if their communication skills are impaired.

Mobility in People with Late-Stage Dementia

As dementia progresses to an advanced stage, the benefits of exercise and rehabilitation may not make a significant difference in improving a resident's mobility. In late-stage dementia, the risk of falling decreases as the resident's functional abilities decline to a point at which he or she must remain in a bed or chair and develops increasing rigidity (Kovach et al., 1997). Ultimately, residents with late-stage dementia become totally dependent and are no longer mobile. Up to this point, however, all possible steps should be taken to address the mobility problems of these residents.

WHAT STAFF CAN DO

Mobility problems are a major issue for long-term care facilities. The yearly cost of care related to falls alone was estimated in 1997 to be $6.8 billion (Verfaille et al., 1997). Beyond the actual direct care costs from these injuries, there are administrative costs and costs relating to the loss of residents' function and decreased quality of life. Knowing that the costs from mobility problems can be so high, addressing these issues should be a priority for long-term care facility staff.

Although mobility problems are not always preventable or treatable, steps can be taken by staff to enhance the functional independence of residents. Taking a therapeutic approach that prioritizes residents' needs over unit schedules can help maximize functional abilities. Using this philosophy, assisting a resident to walk to an activity program is viewed as more important than making a bed on time. This type of therapeutic approach offers important benefits for both residents and staff. It greatly benefits residents with mobility problems because it enables them to more easily maintain their physical conditioning as well as continue their lifestyles and habits. Staff benefit when residents retain higher functional abilities because they require less skilled care.

In long-term care facilities, the personal autonomy of residents with mobility problems too often is compromised. To preserve residents' independence and spirit, facilities should avoid placing restrictions on them. Safety is important, but prioritizing autonomy and freedom can sometimes be more valuable in maintaining residents' quality of life. Thus, staff are constantly faced with making difficult decisions about how to maximize safety while preserving independence. In some situations, these two goals are not compatible, and one must be given priority over the other. Overall, a resident-centered approach that promotes independence as well as the right to take some risks is best. Residents and families also should be given increased opportunities to make some of these difficult care choices themselves. Yet this approach can be a source of great concern for staff, who must provide a safe and therapeutic environment for residents. Therefore, this section discusses a number of approaches that staff can use to help minimize the risk of falling, maintain activity levels, avoid restraints, encourage mobility, and promote and maintain physical conditioning.

Contributors to Resident Falls

Staffing Patterns

In some cases, facility staffing patterns and environmental factors interact to influence rates of fall occurrence. Staff should be aware that many falls happen shortly after a resident moves into a facility. Until new residents become familiar with the environment, they are more likely to fall, and staff should closely monitor their needs and their ability to navigate around the facility. Staff should be aware of the individual risk factors that increase the likelihood of falls and take steps to prevent unnecessary falls from occurring.

When possible, consider placing the residents who need the most assistance in transferring in bedrooms closer to the staff area on the unit. To the greatest extent possible, staff should also plan their schedules based around the daily routines and needs of the residents. If Mrs. McDermott always wakes up at 6 A.M. and needs immediate help getting to the toilet, then staff should build their schedule around being available to help her and other residents like her when they most need assistance. It is not always possible to do this, but staff should be creative and flexible in thinking of ways to address the specific needs of individual residents with mobility problems.

It is logical that more falls occur when there are fewer staff members available to assist residents. Sometimes this problem cannot be helped, but it is important to try to devise innovative solutions. One way to address this issue is to stagger shift changes so that not as many personnel are coming and going at the same time. Typically, staff meet at the beginning of a shift to discuss the conditions of residents. However, this makes them less available to help residents with mobility problems at this time. These residents may then try to perform ADLs (e.g., use the toilet) without assistance and be more prone to falling.

Near Falls

Staff should keep track of "near falls," when residents begin to lose balance but do not fall. It is useful to notice what objects residents commonly grab and assess their stability. For instance, it is better for residents to use grab bars attached to a wall rather than to clutch the backs of chairs. It is often a good idea to observe residents with dementia to determine whether they are having trouble getting around. Being observant and making the environment as safe as possible can help to prevent unnecessary falls. The presence of bruises in a certain location on a resident's body may indicate that he or she is bumping into the same object (e.g., the corner of a dresser) repeatedly. Use this clue to figure out what environmental feature(s) in the room need to be adjusted. (The Behavior Tracking Form in Volume 3, Appendix A can be adapted for this purpose.)

Residents' Fears About Falling

When an older person has experienced a traumatic fall, he or she may be hesitant to participate in certain activities. For example, after Mrs. Lutz falls and breaks her hip while bathing in a tub, she becomes reluctant to take baths and is resistant to staff's interventions. She prefers to take sponge baths for a while rather than using the tub room. (See Chapter 7 for other alternatives to tub baths.) Eventually, she returns to bathing in the tub room, so staff allow extra time for her to get used to being in that setting again and help her to remain calm by reminding her of each step of the bath routine before providing physical assistance. Staff should offer both physical assistance and emotional reassurance every step of the way. There is seldom only one way to do things. Coming up with creative solutions that incorporate residents' preferences not only enhances their quality of life but also can save staff's time and reduces behavior problems such as agitation during ADLs.

When Mobility Becomes Significantly Impaired

Following an injury or surgery, it is important for staff to help residents maintain continuity in their lives. Invite them to go to activities they enjoy and do whatever it takes to help them get there. A wheelchair should be reserved in advance for residents who want to go to the chapel or to a concert. Staff should help them be dressed and ready at the designated time. It is important for people who have experienced a traumatic event such as a fall to be able to look forward to doing something that they enjoy.

Staff should think about what residents with mobility problems *can do* rather than focusing on what they *cannot do*. Some residents may enjoy television, radio, or musical programs. Others may enjoy doing productive tasks such as folding towels and setting tables. Some may enjoy rummaging in boxes filled with buttons or small tool parts. Getting to know each resident's lifelong hobbies and favorite activities can help staff encourage them to continue doing these things. Try to come up with creative solutions to work around mobility problems. Occupational and physical therapy staff may be particularly helpful in designing solutions that meet individual residents' needs.

If a resident is confined to bed following a fall or surgery, bring items from favorite activities to him or her. Take freshly baked cookies to the resident who is normally in the baking group or a bouquet of flowers to someone who walks in the garden everyday. If the resident is used to being outdoors, help him or her to sit near the window so that birds and nature can be seen more easily. Invite a member of the clergy to visit a resident who cannot go to church. Recruit other residents or volunteers to visit and provide companionship to lonely residents. Reassure these residents that they are missed and that others are looking forward to seeing them again soon at activities. Ask both the resident and the family members what will make him or her feel better and then try to provide it. Understand that the resident may be depressed and not feel like doing anything at first.

Mobility problems can be intensely frustrating for residents who are used to being independent. To understand what it feels like to be limited in mobility, staff can try some of the following exercises:

- Put large, heavy rubber bands around your ankles and try to walk around (Figure 3.1)
- Put some beans in your shoes and walk around
- Walk for a significant distance in shoes that are too small or too large

These techniques enable staff to better understand why residents with mobility problems sometimes may unjustly assign blame to others for "letting me fall" or "not helping me." These feelings of frustration often are not directed at staff personally but rather at the situation in which the residents now find

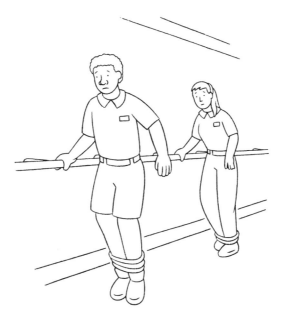

Figure 3.1.   Put large, heavy rubber bands around
your ankles and try to walk around.

themselves. Staff should be patient and validate the residents' feelings. Doing small, thoughtful things can really make a difference in improving the residents' quality of life after an injury or surgery. Furthermore, this helps renew trust and build rapport.

Help residents set attainable goals for returning to former activities. When a resident is physically ready, encourage him or her to become mobile again. Especially after an injury, people are more likely to fall again if they are anxious and develop a hesitant or irregular gait when walking. Some family members and caregivers may become overprotective of residents with mobility problems, especially when their physical conditions suggest that they may be prone to fall repeatedly. These residents are sensitive to the feelings that other people are projecting. If they are treated as frail or incompetent, then they are more likely to become that way. Therefore, it is important to avoid creating a fear of falling in residents whenever possible. Encourage them to continue to be active and not withdraw socially.

Truth About Restraints

In the past, many staff members typically relied on restraints to enhance resident safety. However, there are numerous negative physical, psychological, and social consequences to restraint usage for residents. In addition, using restraints also has a negative impact on relationships between staff and residents by damaging trust and rapport. Every time staff consider restraining a resident, they should imagine that it is one of their own family members or themselves and consider how they would feel then about using the restraint. To further increase staff sensitivity, try the following exercise during an in-service program: Have staff members place various types of restraints on other staff members and let them experience what it actually feels like to be restrained for several hours.

Educating Staff About Alternatives to Restraint Use

Staff need to be educated about alternatives to using restraints to understand that there are other effective options. The first step is educating staff about how mechanical and chemical restraints have been overused and about their drawbacks. Review the policies at your facility and form a committee that monitors this issue on an ongoing basis. This committee should keep up with the literature on alternatives to restraint usage. For example, Braun and Lipson (1993) made a strong case that the only time that a restraint should even be considered is when resident or caregiver safety is at high risk, medical treatment is compromised, or all other alternatives have been exhausted. They stated that enhancement of safety, fall prevention, and illness are not sufficient reasons for consistently using physical restraints with residents. Because of the negative consequences of restraint use, these authors highly recommended that all facilities implement a restraint-free policy or a restraint reduction program.

Good education programs teach staff to understand why restraints are not the best solution and to support the use of a restraint-free approach. A restraint-free environment should be presented to staff as being more therapeutic for residents and be continually emphasized. Staff must be encouraged to think creatively about strategies other than restraint use. Staff should be reassured that instituting a restraint reduction program will not result in a higher likelihood of them being accused of negligence if a resident should fall or become injured while in their care. Although some facilities justify restraint use by stating that the facility could be liable if an unrestrained resident becomes injured, this fear is largely unfounded. Indeed, several studies have found that long-term care facilities were more likely to be sued by families whose relative suffered injury as a result of being restrained than by the families of residents who fell while unrestrained (Epstein, 1994; Tideiksaar, 1998).

Relationship of Staffing Level to Restraint Use

It is often assumed that there is a relationship between the number of staff and the level of restraint use in a facility. However, it is a mistaken belief that a low staff-to-resident ratio makes restraints necessary for providing good care. Actually, to use restraints properly requires a higher staff-to-resident ratio. Otherwise, there will not be enough staff to attend to restrained residents, check on them, and provide appropriate exercise. Although restraining residents may seem to be a quicker and easier way to provide care, residents who are regularly restrained will develop greater immobility from inactivity. This will make them more dependent on skilled care from staff. Along with their physical deconditioning, they may become more resistant to medical care and demonstrate behavior problems commonly associated with restraint use, including increased agitation and paranoia.

Reducing the Need for Restraint Use

Restraints should never be used by staff as a way to supervise residents. Family members, friends, volunteers, and others can make excellent companions to sit with residents so that they do not need to be restrained. When residents are bored, they are more likely to wander around, possibly placing them at an increased risk for falling. Designing a good ongoing structured activity program with group as well as one-to-one activities helps residents to stay busy. If the facility can recruit volunteers to help escort more independent residents to certain activities, then staff will be able to spend more time helping more frail residents to walk to these events.

Both staff and families should be involved in the decision to remove restraints. Families often feel that the freedom and happiness of their loved one supersedes the risk of falling, but this is an individual choice that families are best qualified to make. Staff should educate families regarding the pros and cons of each approach rather than dictate what should be done. To prevent legal problems, the facility should institute a standard protocol for explaining the resident's level of risk for falling to family members. Ask them (or the resident, if he or she is competent) to sign a written statement expressing their preferences regarding the use of restraints. This issue should be reviewed periodically as residents' conditions change or they become more frail over time. Families appreciate a facility's proactive stance on this issue and the good care that their loved one is receiving at the facility.

Residents should be prepared properly for restraint removal so that the process will be safe and therapeutic for them. For each resident involved in a restraint reduction program, staff should create a series of appropriate goals and chart them in the resident's care plan. These goals might include implementing a daily walking schedule to improve gait and weight-bearing ability, or devising a suitable toileting schedule and ensuring that staff are available to assist the resident as needed. Staff should be trained to assist residents with mobility problems in performing their ADLs and any high-risk activities rather than automatically doing these activities for them. If these residents' rooms are located near staff areas, then they can receive help and be observed more easily. Remind the residents to ask for help when they get up, and provide them with frequent cues to use mobility aids and assistive devices. Residents should be made comfortable and their physical needs attended to promptly so that they do not fall when trying to take care of their needs without staff assistance.

Mobility Aids

Staff can provide different types of mobility aids to help residents in maintaining independence and minimizing excess disability. Mobility aids include canes, walkers, wheelchairs, and certain types of bathroom equipment (see "Where to Find Products" later in this chapter for sources). Many older people do not realize the difference that such devices make in both reducing their physical fatigue and helping them to get around. Mobility aids also enable residents to conserve energy for activities that they really enjoy doing.

Social Stigma Associated with Mobility Aids

Some older people perceive a social stigma associated with using a mobility aid. They may fear that others will view them as frail if they are using a cane or a walker. Some residents may feel differently about using a mobility aid on a temporary basis (e.g., after a hip fracture) rather than permanently. When residents are embarrassed, they may conceal the mobility aid out of sight and out of reach (e.g., behind a door). In certain cases, they may be vague about where they put the device and claim that it is not necessary ("Oh, it's around here somewhere, but I can get around in my room without it"). Therefore, staff may need to brainstorm an effective strategy to encourage residents to use their mobility aids. Staff can enhance the functionality of the device; for example, a bag can be attached to a walker or wheelchair in which the resident can carry possessions such as tissues, candy, or eyeglasses. Another option is to make a bag that can be tied around the resident's waist, somewhat like a "fanny pack." Finally, the device can be made more attractive to the resident (e.g., a cane can be painted purple if that is the resident's favorite color).

When residents are hesitant about using mobility aids, it is important for staff to validate their feelings. Staff always should be positive about using mobility aids and treat them as "tools for living" rather than "aids for the declining" (Rush & Ouellet, 1997). Praise residents when they use mobility aids in ways that promote their functional independence (Figure 3.2). Point out how the aid helps them complete tasks on their own that might otherwise take a long time to accomplish. For example, a resident using a walker can get to an activity program in half the time and be more safe and less fatigued when he or she arrives, and therefore be able to enjoy the program.

Mobility Aids for Residents with Dementia

Getting residents with dementia to accept and regularly use mobility aids can be challenging. Studies have shown that people with dementia use fewer mobility aids and have a higher rate of dissatisfaction with them (e.g., Rush & Ouellet, 1997). Some residents with dementia may be unaware that they need a mobility aid because they compensate by holding onto walls, furniture, or other objects in the environment. Staff need to be observant so that they can determine whether these residents would benefit from mobility aids.

Using a mobility aid is an adjustment for all older adults but can be particularly difficult for someone with memory impairment. Most people do not

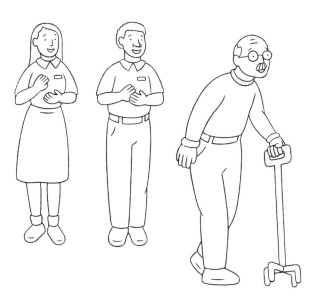

Figure 3.2.   Praise residents when they use mobility aids in ways that promote their functional independence.

Table 3.1. Types of canes and walkers

	Description	Pros	Cons
Canes			
Single-tipped	Simplest type of mobility aid; helps with supporting body weight instead of relying on lower extremities; can be made of wood, fiberglass, or aluminum	Supports some body weight and is easy to use and transport	Not as much support as some other types of mobility aids
Quad	Has a pedestal base with four feet for extra support	Provides more support	Less cosmetically appealing
Walkers			
Hemiwalker	Prescribed in some cases to reduce lateral instability	More compact than pickup walker	Not appropriate in all situations
Pickup	Provides a wider base of support than the hemiwalker	Increases lateral stability	Residents with dementia may have trouble learning the sequence of steps required to use a pickup walker correctly
Gliding	Has plastic glides rather than rubber tips (e.g., pickup walker) attached to the bases of the legs	Can be easier to operate than pickup walker	Only for use on smooth, flat floors (e.g., linoleum); when using this walker on carpet or other uneven floor surfaces with boundaries, it will stop completely or tip over when the surface changes
Rolling	Can be pushed instead of picked up off the ground; some models feature hand brakes	Can be used on carpeted surfaces	Less sturdy and stable than pickup walker

grips, can influence whether the resident is able to use it successfully. A walker that is too heavy may be difficult for a resident to lift and move forward, whereas a walker that is too light may not provide adequate balance and support. The device must be positioned at a height that ensures maximum comfort and safety for the resident. Positioning a walker frame too high can lead to problems such as arm and shoulder fatigue, incorrect posture, and poor balance. Positioning a walker frame too low can cause a resident to bend over too far to use it, and the resident may actually fall forward over the stringer bar (the horizontal bar at the front of the walker) when walking.

Walkers sometimes can be difficult to use in space-limited areas, although this should not be a problem in most newer facilities. Residents are less likely to use walkers when they are difficult to navigate in a small space. For example, residents with narrow bedrooms may find it easier to grab on to walls or chairs rather than using their walkers. Similarly, in public spaces they may be less inclined to use their walkers when there are no places to easily "park" these devices (e.g., when there are many walkers in the dining room at mealtimes). "What the Environment Can Do" provides a more extensive explanation of how to make various rooms more user friendly for residents with mobility problems.

Wheelchairs can give mobility to a person who is unable to ambulate independently. Selecting the correct wheelchair and good wheelchair positioning are two critical elements for safety and maximizing functional ability. Wheelchairs should be individually fitted both for size and specific features, including seat width, depth, height, footrests, back support, armrests, and tray tables. In addition, some safety concerns are specific to the use of wheelchairs by residents with dementia. For example, they may have difficulty remembering to lock the brakes before attempting to rise from a wheelchair, and if they lean forward to pick things up from the ground, they may tumble out of a wheelchair.

Exercise to Promote and Maintain Physical Conditioning

Staff should encourage residents with mobility problems to participate in regular exercise programs at a level that is appropriate for each individual. (Remember, however, that before any resident begins an exercise program, he or she should consult a doctor.) Even low levels of exercise produce modest improvements that can increase functional ability. It is never too late to start exercising. For residents who do not have a history of being physically active, staff should try to find simple, easy exercises that they can do to preserve their remaining abilities. Tailor the exercise program toward addressing residents' specific physical impairments. A multidisciplinary approach involving the resident's doctor, nursing, physical therapy, occupational therapy, and activities staff is necessary in designing exercise programs that best meet the needs of different types of residents.

Many different styles of exercises, including wheelchair or armchair aerobics, can be beneficial for residents. Activities that are unrealistic or juvenile should be avoided. Some activities that emphasize gross motor skills, such as tossing a big beach ball or waving a parachute, are unfamiliar and not meaningful to residents. Exercises such as those that residents might have done at home on a daily basis (e.g., simple stretching exercises) are best. And, exercise need not always occur in a structured program. Some people may enjoy familiar tasks that inherently involve exercise, such as light housecleaning or gardening.

Sports and forms of exercise that were part of residents' lives before moving to a nursing facility often can be incorporated into exercise programs. A facility in Wisconsin built a bowling alley because this sport had been a lifelong activity for many residents. A dance hall atmosphere can be created for residents who enjoy ballroom dancing. Staff should try to provide activities in which residents can show their competence from many years of experience and a chance to show off their special abilities (e.g., Larry's famous golf swing). These skills have been an important part of their identities for a long time, so if residents become frustrated by the limitations that illness places on their performance, then staff should be supportive. They should acknowledge the losses that residents experience and encourage them to continue, but also understand and respect residents' decisions not to participate because they believe they cannot maintain their previous level of expertise. Staff can help them find new activities.

Staff should closely monitor the physical performance of residents as they exercise. Sessions should be shorter when the weather is hot or air quality is poor. Consistency in staffing will help ensure that the physical limits of individual residents are not exceeded. Remind residents to stop exercising immediately if they feel pain. People with dementia may not always recognize when they are overstraining or doing something that will cause pain later. Residents who cannot communicate well may not be able to tell staff members that they are feeling pain. Staff should watch the residents' facial expressions closely; if residents are grimacing or appear to be in pain, staff should intervene so that residents are not injured further.

Exercise equipment must be adapted to each resident's needs. A Nerf ball or beach ball can be used instead of a regulation basketball, which is heavier. Also, adequate room must be available to accommodate exercising residents so that they do not become injured during an activity. In general, residents should be at least one arm's length apart before starting the activity. Objects that are being tossed should be kept low and away from residents' faces. Set up the room so that residents can see and hear well during the activity.

Residents should be proactive in shaping the exercise program, such as choosing the music for dancing or picking the color for the bowling team's shirts. Staff can take pictures of the residents while they exercise so that the pictures can be enjoyed later. If residents are capable of being competitive and enjoying competition, then reward their participation by, for example, making a list of the best bowling scores and hanging it on the wall. Do not force residents with dementia to perform competitively or put extra pressure on them if they are not interested or react with hostility.

Difference Staff Can Make in Successful Rehabilitation

Staff can play a major role in supporting residents with mobility problems who are involved in rehabilitation. Staff should reward residents' success in rehabilitation with lots of encouragement and praise. When you see residents in the hallway, compliment them on how well they are walking, standing, or using a cane, as appropriate. Even if residents with dementia do not fully understand, they will pick up on your positive sentiment. Small extras such as giving residents a greeting card congratulating them when they make progress in rehabilitation can make a big difference.

Staff should promote the use of the skills learned from rehabilitation throughout the day. When a resident routinely does certain activities in therapy but does not do them at other times during the day, analyze how these activities can be incorporated into his or her daily routine. Break tasks such as ADLs into steps and determine which steps the resident could do independently or with minimal assistance. Cues (e.g., verbal directions, picture cards) can be provided to help him or her accomplish these steps. If a resident is motivated to go to a favorite activity program, then he or she should be encouraged to walk there with staff assistance rather than going in a wheelchair. Finding the few extra minutes to do this can be beneficial for the resident. As mentioned, staff should be trained to prioritize this type of therapeutic interaction; it is often far more important than maintaining the unit's daily schedule. Staff also should talk with each other at shift changes about what each resident has done that day and assess his or her level of fatigue. If residents already have pushed themselves to the limit physically and they are encouraged to do more, then there may be a catastrophic reaction.

Residents who are depressed may not want to expend the energy that is required to participate in the rehabilitation process. In this case, staff should tailor the rehabilitation program to meet the residents' needs. For example, schedule therapy at a time of day when they have the most energy and are in a receptive mood. Learn about their lifelong patterns—if a resident is a morning person, hold his or her therapy session right after breakfast. Staff need to be flexible and recognize that, like themselves, residents may feel better or worse on particular days. When residents do not sleep well during the night, they may not feel like participating in therapy the next morning because they are tired. On a rainy day they may feel achy and have more pain than usual. Always listen to the residents and let them express their feelings and preferences regarding participation. Do not try to force them to comply, but instead offer positive encouragement and support.

Staff should make sure that therapy does not conflict with other activities that are important to residents (e.g., a favorite bingo game). These scheduling conflicts may make them hostile to the therapy process, which is counterproductive. Reassure residents that going to therapy (particularly if it is located off the unit) does not mean that they will miss meals or other important events such as family visits. Residents can be allowed to bring certain items (e.g., a purse) that they are worried about leaving behind to the therapy session. When they return to the unit, give them positive reinforcement for going to rehabilitation and working on skills that will help them be more independent.

WHAT THE ENVIRONMENT CAN DO

As we age, we may rely on the environment for even more support but may not be able to manipulate it as easily as we did when we were younger. Environmental modifications that promote independent mobility and reduce the risk of injury are a worthwhile investment. When environments are hard to navigate, residents with mobility problems are more likely to fall. In addition, residents with excess disability often require greater staff assistance. Even facilities built for older adults do not automatically support maximum mobility. A facility should begin by looking at its whole environment to determine how difficult it is for residents with mobility problems to function. An architect or interior designer is not necessary to begin making improvements to a facility. All people regularly make changes to improve their environment, such as adjusting a window blind to avoid glare or moving a piece of furniture out of the way. The following environmental modifications are related to maximizing resident mobility:

- Providing appropriate lighting and decreasing glare
- Using appropriate flooring surfaces and treatments
- Making use of color and pattern
- Optimizing furniture and furniture arrangement
- Providing appropriate handrails
- Supplying communication devices for staff

The remainder of this section is divided into two subsections. The first looks at how these modifications can affect residents' mobility; the second looks at these issues in relationship to specific spaces in the facility.

Environmental Aspects that Support Mobility

Lighting and Glare

Good lighting throughout a facility is essential. Lighting helps residents to navigate their environment and reduces excess disability. When there is low illumination, residents are more likely to have trouble perceiving subtle differences between objects in the environment (e.g., the threshold of a door). These problems increase the risk of falls. Furthermore, residents can become disoriented and upset when they cannot see where they are going or cannot see obstacles in their path. Lighting levels need to be higher for an older person to see as well as a younger person sees. However, light levels must be increased carefully because they can contribute to glare conditions to which many residents are sensitive. Lighting levels also need to be consistent. As eyes age, they can no longer adjust rapidly to varying lighting conditions. Some people may be blinded temporarily by sudden changes of light levels. As a result, they may be at a greater risk of falling.

A resident's ability to navigate in the environment is also inhibited by direct glare coming from windows and unshielded bulbs. Indirect glare from reflective surfaces such as highly polished floors also causes problems. In particular, floor glare negatively affects mobility because, with it, residents often cannot judge changes in ground elevation. People with poor vision, dementia, or both may interpret highly polished floors as being slippery or as having puddles. As a result, they may adjust their gait, which can lead to falls.

Floor Surfaces and Floor Treatments

Floor surfaces need to be nonslip and need to have low drag resistance (where the surface has less friction) for residents who use assistive devices. Both carpeting and resilient flooring (e.g., vinyl) have benefits and drawbacks. Although resilient flooring has less drag, it also is easier to slip and fall on it. Carpeting provides higher drag for people who use a wheelchair or who shuffle their feet, and it is more slip resistant.

Certain types of shoes, specifically the material of the soles, are more appropriate for certain flooring materials. Shoes with more grip (e.g., tennis shoes, shoes with crepe soles) provide more traction on resilient flooring than do shoes with leather or plastic soles. Conversely, rubber or crepe soles are more likely to catch on carpeting and cause residents to lose their balance and fall, particularly residents who tend to shuffle their feet when they walk. However, research suggests that, although there may be more falls on carpeting, there are fewer and less serious injuries associated with these falls than with falls on resilient flooring (Wise, 1996). Falls are more likely to occur at transition points (real or perceived), that is, at transitions from resilient flooring to carpeting or where there are sharp contrasts in floor coloring (e.g., between the border and the field of a hallway carpet).

When replacing flooring in a particular area, each facility must decide which type of floor is best suited for its residents, keeping all of the issues mentioned above in mind (see "What the Environment Can Do" in Chapter 5 for a comparison of carpeting and resilient floors). Regardless of floor type, floor surfaces must be level. Poor depth perception can make it hard for older people to judge floor transitions when walking. Gentle transitions provide fewer barriers for residents and reduce the chance of tripping and hence falling.

Color and Pattern

The color and pattern of a surface can either aid mobility or hinder it. Color contrast can be used to help define the edges of items so that residents can clearly see where to sit or grab on to an object. Lack of color contrast or the use of color contrast in the wrong place can make residents stumble or fall. Patterned or contrasting floor surfaces may appear to older adults as raised or lowered surfaces instead of flat ground (Figure 3.4). This phenomenon is called *visual cliffing*. Visual cliffing may cause residents to try to step over these surfaces or to avoid walking on them. It may not be possible for a facility to change the flooring immediately, but this discussion of appropriate colors and patterns should be kept in mind for future changes in flooring.

Furniture and Furniture Arrangement

Furniture should be selected on the basis of how well it supports residents' needs and its attractiveness. Furniture ordered from a health care company is not necessarily designed to be supportive of the residents of a long-term care facility. Furniture companies frequently repackage typical hospitality furniture for the health care market. They often emphasize cleanability and durability rather than proper support or ease of use. Furniture also must be arranged in an appropriate manner to be supportive for residents. Too much

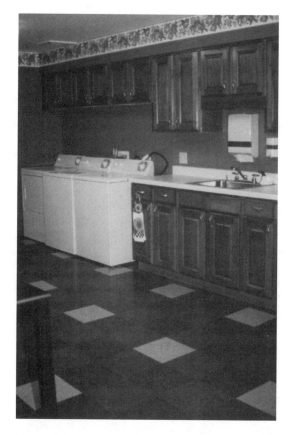

Figure 3.4. Patterned floor surfaces may produce *visual cliffing*, which looks like raised or lowered surfaces.

furniture can be difficult to maneuver around, and not enough may make it difficult for a resident to find a place to sit.

Handrails

The appropriate handrails can be critical to providing assistive support for residents. Some residents in wheelchairs use handrails to pull themselves down the hall. Others who walk will use handrails to lean against to rest or to maintain balance. Because each of these uses requires a different type of handrail, the installation of handrails requires careful consideration. Handrails must be appropriately shaped, easily recognizable, and placed in appropriate locations. A full discussion of handrails is provided in "Improving Mobility in Specific Areas."

Communication Devices

Effective communication is necessary for staff to provide adequate support for residents with mobility problems. A nurse call light does not indicate what is needed or who the respondent should be. Many facilities lack two-way communication between the staff station and the residents' rooms. This means that staff cannot call for additional assistance. Frequently, the wrong staff member is sent to respond to a call, and more staff time is wasted finding the appropriate staff member to respond. In addition, staff may be forced to rely on an public address system, which contributes unnecessary noise on the unit. There are a variety of products that facilitate communication among staff and help to maintain a quiet environment. Systems are also available that alert staff when residents are at risk for falling. A cord is attached to residents' clothing; when they try to stand up or get out of bed, the other end of the cord pulls away from the alarm monitor, and an alarm sounds.

Improving Mobility in Specific Areas

The environmental factors discussed previously can be manipulated in a variety of ways to improve residents' mobility. Staff should observe how residents are getting around in specific areas and, when barriers are identified, think about creative ways to eliminate them. Special attention should be directed to observing how residents maneuver in their bedrooms and bathrooms. The residents' daily routines and whether the physical environment complements their needs should be considered. For example, when a resident cannot easily get from sitting in a favorite chair to the bathroom, determine what features in the environment can be altered to make this route less difficult to navigate. This can be done using the 5 Ws—who, what [e.g., what behavior], where, when, and why—part of the behavior tracking process that is described in Volume 3, Chapter 1. To use the 5 Ws with regard to mobility, staff should think about who is having these difficulties and why they are occurring—What is present in the environment (e.g., furniture) that makes it hard for residents to get around? What is in the area that residents might grab on to for support? In which areas are residents most likely to stumble or fall? When do specific residents with mobility problems experience the most trouble (e.g., at night when the room is dark and they are tired)? This section looks in more detail at how each of these issues affects mobility in specific areas in the unit.

Hallways

Lighting and Glare

Long hallways with poor lighting are typical in many older facilities. Because fluorescent ceiling-mounted light fixtures are frequently seen from a distance in a hallway, controlling side glare is an important feature. Some fluorescent light fixtures that are not recessed in a ceiling grid emit light from the sides, which results in side glare. These fixtures are referred to as *wrap-around fixtures* and should be avoided if possible. If your facility is already fitted with these fixtures, the fixture manufacturer may be able to provide replacement covers with solid (opaque) sides.

Hallway lighting should include indirect lighting techniques as much as possible. It is important to light not only the floor surface but the wall surfaces as well. Residents may not be able to see handrails or door signs if only the center of the hall is lit well. Fixtures should be spaced appropriately to provide even lighting of at least 30 footcandles (see "What the Environment Can Do" in Volume 1, Chapter 2 for an explanation of footcandles).

Strategies to improve lighting can be implemented over time so that they can fit into your facility's budget. Newer light fixtures are frequently more energy efficient, and thus pay for themselves over time. Facility personnel should assess hallway lighting, looking for dim lighting, harsh lighting, or lighting that causes excessive glare. Louvered diffusers that distribute light evenly can replace the standard recessed fluorescent lights in a ceiling grid found in many facilities. These diffusers reduce side glare but also darken the ceiling. To help increase hallway lighting levels, facility personnel should consider installing Americans with Disabilities Act (ADA)–compliant wall sconces to indirectly illuminate the hallway walls (see "Where to Find Products" at the end of this chapter). Sconces should not use exposed bulbs. In addition, the light from sconces should be directed both up and down the walls.

Facilities that are planning to replace ceiling fixtures should consider purchasing parabolic fixtures that have a built-in diffuser to reduce side glare (Figure 3.5). The smaller grids reduce the amount of glare near the fixtures. When installing indirect lighting to avoid glare, consider installing indirect fluorescent up-and-down lights along the walls. These fixtures spread the light across the walls and the ceiling surface to light the hallway. It may be more expensive to install wall-mounted fixtures in existing buildings. ADA requires that all wall-mounted fixtures extend not more than 4 inches into the hallway unless these fixtures are mounted 80 inches above the floor. Facilities with a ceiling height of less than 8 feet should use ADA–compliant wall fixtures. Those with a ceiling height of more than 8 feet may be able to use a ceiling-

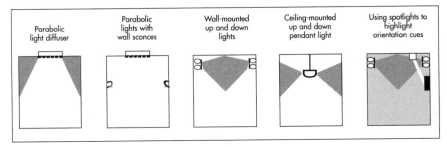

Figure 3.5.   Different types of lighting conditions in hallways can be provided by various light fixtures.

mounted indirect up-and-down light fixture to illuminate the hallways. If primarily indirect lighting is used to illuminate the halls, then highlight landmarks, interesting features, or signage with direct spot lighting.

Glare can create visual distortions that can contribute to gait disturbances and falls. There are several common causes of glare in hallways. First, facilities often have resilient floor surfaces in the halls that are polished frequently. These floors reflect any intense light, causing glare. Second, often there are abrupt changes in lighting levels in hallways. For example, strong light may be coming through a window or door at the end of the hall that leads outside. This light can be blinding ("glare hotspots"; Figure 3.6). Third, windows in residents' rooms with no window treatments may permit light to come in through doorways, and this creates unexpected glare on floors. Finally, light emanating from hallways that open on to lounges can also create a sudden increase in lighting levels in the hall. Every facility should review its hallways for glare hotspots. Take a photograph of the hallways during the daytime. When you look at the developed photo, you may see glare hotspots that were not evident previously.

Cover windows along hallways or at the ends of hallways where glare is the most prominent with sheer curtains or draperies. Curtains should be installed on windows with an eastern or western exposure, because sunlight is more intense and lower in the sky during the morning and afternoon. Blinds should not be used in hallway windows because they can create alternating light and dark slits, which are disturbing especially to people with dementia, and they create distorted patterns on the floor. By using window treatments, you may feel that you are blocking the light in these halls, but you are actually making it easier for residents to get around.

There are two main solutions to reflected glare on a floor. A more expensive solution is replacing the flooring with a material that does not cause

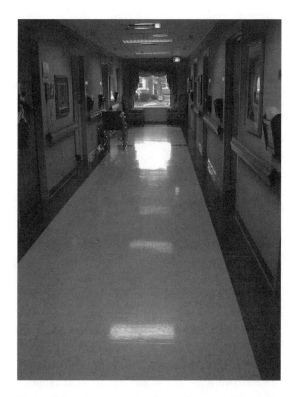

Figure 3.6.   An example of glare hotspots. Visual distortion is caused by glare from both a door at the end of a hallway and light from ceiling fixtures reflected on a polished floor surface.

glare (see the following discussion). The low-cost solution is to avoid polishing the floor. A pervasive although false belief is that a shiny floor must be a clean floor. However, a floor can be clean without being shiny. Shiny floors require extra maintenance and can reflect light, causing glare. If your facility is concerned that family members may complain because they will think cleanliness standards are falling, administrators can send a letter or hang a notice in the lobby explaining that the floors are not being polished because glare disturbs the residents. Most floors do require a sealer coat to maintain their appearance. Ask the maintenance department to find a sealer with a matte finish that does not require a polish coat. Sometimes a polish can be buffed with a blue pad to reduce the amount of shine. Because each flooring material has different maintenance requirements and warranties, the flooring manufacturer's representative should be contacted to determine the best way to reduce the floor's luster.

Flooring

When selecting flooring, the facility should keep mobility issues in mind (see "Where to Find Products" at the end of this chapter for flooring sources). In many cases, carpeting is a good option. Not only does it not reflect glare but it also cushions falls, absorbs sound, and gives the facility a more homelike appearance. Carpeting can be less costly and time consuming than tile or linoleum to maintain. One drawback to carpeting is the drag on the feet of residents who walk with a shuffling gait or use mobility devices. Low-pile or loop-pile carpeting minimizes this effect. Textured resilient floor surfaces can provide traction, which helps reduce slipping. Some resilient flooring does not require polish or sealers, which increase maintenance costs and glare. Such products may have to be replaced more frequently than regular floor-ing; replacement costs should be carefully weighed against the eventual sav-ings in maintenance costs and the well-being of residents. Texture-coated flooring that is designed to diffuse light and reduce glare is more expensive than regular resilient flooring, but it does not have to be replaced as often.

Transitions between floor surfaces in hallway doors and openings should be reviewed carefully. A transition usually occurs when flooring types change, such as vinyl to carpet (this frequently occurs in residents' bedroom doorways). The two floor surfaces should be as level with each other as possi-ble. A metal or plastic transition strip is usually installed. These strips are ob-stacles to wheelchairs or walkers, especially when the residents who use them have limited strength. Transition strips should be beveled to provide a gentle incline when floor surfaces change. ADA requires that these strips not exceed ½ inch in height, and strips that are more than ¼ inch in height should be beveled at a slope of 1:2. Johnsonite is one of the first manufacturers to make a vinyl transition strip for carpet to vinyl that meets ADA standards (see "Where to Find Products" at the end of the chapter). Tracks for sliding doors and automatic doors also should be reviewed to ensure that residents can move through these openings easily.

Color and Pattern

Appropriate color and pattern must be used on the walls and floors of every hallway. Wallcoverings with bold patterns that appear to move or can distract attention from landmarks or signage in the halls should be avoided. Realistic-looking, full-height wall murals should be avoided because they can lead to confusion among residents as to where the wall stops and the mural begins. Materials used on the walls should have a matte finish to avoid reflecting light. The color of the hallway floor should contrast with the walls to provide a clear delineation. Avoid the use of a carpeted wall base that blurs the transition between the wall and the floor. The color of the wall base should match the wall, not the floor. A patterned carpet hides stains more effectively, but the pattern must be chosen carefully. Carpet patterns should not be excessively busy or have strongly contrasting colors. Darker areas may resemble a depression while lighter areas may look raised. Residents may stumble thinking that they are changing levels or trying to step over a perceived hole in the floor. Borders should be avoided unless the color of both the border and the field are the same intensity and hue. A black-and-white photograph or a photocopied sample of the carpet, border, or both will clarify whether the colors in the pattern create the illusion of a change in level.

Furniture

Long hallways are hard for residents with mobility problems to navigate. Whenever possible, seating options along the length of the hallway should be incorporated so that, if residents become tired, they can sit down to rest. (A balance must be maintained between keeping the hallway clear for residents to easily navigate its length and creating appropriate rest stops, however.) When residents know that these seating options are available, they may be more willing to try to walk to an activity program or the dining room. The local fire marshal can determine whether there are locations along the hallway where furniture can be placed (see Figure 2.2). Try to locate chairs strategically so that they break up the tunnel-like appearance of some hallways. Of course, too many items in a hall can also create problems. Keep equipment and clutter out of hallways to enable residents to easily see what is ahead. Also, keep residents' use of handrails in mind when creating rest areas. Try to provide a complete handrail on at least one side of each hallway.

Handrails

It may be hard for residents with dementia to figure out the purpose of handrails because they are neither familiar nor homelike. Yet they are important safety features for residents with mobility problems, especially those who often forget to use their mobility aids. Although the design trend in the early 21st century is to visually blend the handrail into the wall, this practice may make it difficult for residents with dementia or impaired vision to find the handrail.

Appropriate handrail shape is also important. Handrails should be round on top where the hand will grasp the rail. The acceptable diameter of the gripping surface is between 1¼ and 1½ inches. The space between the wall and the handrail should be 1½ inches to avoid the danger of a person's arm being caught behind the rail during a fall. The ends of all handrails should curve back toward the wall so a resident's body or clothing cannot get caught on a handrail when he or she is walking close to the wall.

The height of handrails also can be an issue. Wheelchair users may find that a low rail height of 36 inches works best for their needs when pulling their wheelchairs along a corridor. Ambulatory residents who may use a handrail as a resting and steadying point require a height of 41 inches (Hiatt, 1991). Each facility should look at its population to determine which height to choose, and each also should investigate whether the state mandates a handrail height. Both features can be provided by incorporating a leaning rail and a handrail (Figure 3.7). A leaning rail is a decorative molding placed above the handrail that residents can use to lean against.

If your facility's handrails do not comply with the standards mentioned above, then consider retrofitting or replacing them. Wood handrails can sometimes be recut to proper dimensions or replaced with new rails and then rehung on the same brackets.

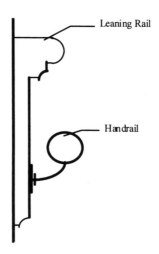

Figure 3.7. An example of a combination of leaning rails and handrails.

Communication Devices

Residents who require mobility assistance rely on staff being in the right location. Effective staff communication can support resident mobility. Systems that have been used to improve communication between businesses also can work inside a long-term care facility (see "Where to Find Products" for sources). Staff members who are needed frequently can carry cellular phones. Portable paging systems also can provide a means of communicating without using public address systems, which can be disruptive to residents. Pagers with liquid crystal displays can provide additional information about which resident called or who is needed. This means that staff spend less time responding to calls intended for someone other than themselves and more time assisting residents. A paging system sometimes can be added to a new nurse call system. Some nurse call systems are equipped with lights that can be color coded to indicate staff types, so the proper assistance is sent the first time.

Residents' Rooms and Public Areas

Lighting and Glare

Bedroom lighting in long-term care facilities frequently is limited to an over-the-bed light and a light in the entry area. Most regulating agencies require a high light level above the bed pillow, but this assumes that residents spend most of their time in bed. These lights rarely completely light a room. Also, because frequently the controls for over-the-bed lights are located by the bed, residents must walk into a dark room and over to the bed to turn on a light. A favorite chair or other area where the resident spends considerable time in the room also should be lit well for easy transfer. Some residents cannot remember to turn light switches on and off. A good solution is a light that is controlled by a motion sensor. Installing a night-light to help residents' eyes adjust gradually can help alleviate night blindness. The facility should review the use of night-lights with respect to each resident because some residents may interpret shadows inappropriately and become frightened.

Overhead direct lighting is used most commonly in public spaces. In areas used by residents to perform certain tasks or to participate in activities, these lights can be supplemented with table and floor lamps. Lighting levels must be consistent in areas where there are subtle changes in levels or materials that might cause residents to stumble. Glare from windows in both bedrooms and public areas must be controlled. Walking from a darker corridor into a brightly lit room with open curtains can cause temporary blindness. To filter strong light, a sheer window treatment or curtains can be installed. Avoid the use of metal or plastic blinds, which can create a confusing pattern on the floor and do not completely filter light.

Flooring

In residents' bedrooms, flooring should be slip resistant and should not contribute to glare. Carpeting is a great choice. It needs less maintenance than bare floors, which means caring for it may disturb residents less often. However, some carpet-cleaning equipment is noisier than the cleaning methods that are used on resilient flooring (see "Where to Find Products" for sources of quiet vacuum cleaners). Compared with a hard surface, carpeting can cushion a resident's fall. Staff should make sure that the transition from carpeting to any hard surface is beveled and does not exceed ¼ inch without installing a small ramp. Nonslip strips can be applied in multiple locations in a facility to enhance residents' safety. For example, in residents' bedrooms, the strips can be used in front of beds to provide greater stability. Vinyl floors that do not require polishing or have a matte appearance are also a good choice.

Color and Pattern

Color should be used to highlight the contrast between objects in the environment because residents may have difficulty transferring when they cannot see the edges of objects well. Make sure that bedroom chairs and bedspreads contrast with the floor's surface. View fabric samples through a piece of yellow acetate (available in art supply stores) to simulate the vision of an older adult. The contrast between the floor and the bedspread or chair cover should still be obvious through the acetate. The use of patterns on walls and furniture in bedrooms and living rooms is more acceptable because it is familiar, but you must still be careful in your selection. A pattern with subtle repeats is best; large stripes that resemble bars should be avoided. Also, avoid using patterns behind displays of residents' personal items or signs that you wish them to see clearly.

Furniture

Residents commonly use furniture for support when transferring and walking. Staff should make sure that all of the furniture in the facility is stable. No piece of furniture should give way when residents lean against it. Furniture should be arranged so that it suits the needs of individual residents. For example, residents with Parkinson's disease benefit from open space in their rooms. These residents typically have difficulties, once in motion, in slowing down to change direction and move around furniture. Conversely, residents with arthritis may do better with furniture that is arranged close together so that they can hold onto it for support.

Some residents may be ambulatory but unsteady, which is a cause for concern when they try to walk unaided. Some types of seating discourage residents from trying to get up and walk without assistance. Deep-seated or soft-cushioned chairs or recliners can be used for this purpose. Another option is to place a wedge cushion on a chair seat with the widest part of the cushion placed at the front of the chair. Because these nonmechanical restraints allow residents to shift more easily in their seats, they are less likely to get pressure sores. There are also chair alarms that function similarly to the bed alarm system described in "Communication Devices." Technically, these seating alternatives are restraints, but they may be much more acceptable to residents and their families. These options successfully avoid the visual stigma of residents' appearing to be tied down. Residents are likely to exhibit fewer behavioral problems, such as combativeness and agitation, with their use.

Many falls in nursing facilities occur during transfers in and out of bed. Support rails can be added to beds to provide assistance while a resident transfers to and from the bed. Although bed siderails enable residents to make safe bed transfers, they are often used in long-term care facilities to prevent residents from rolling out of bed. However, residents who try to get out of a bed with siderails without assistance may be more likely to fall. When residents climb over elevated bedrails, their arms and legs can get caught in the rails, which greatly increases their risk of being injured. Climbing over bedrails also results in falling from a greater height, usually onto a hard floor surface, increasing the risk of fractures and head trauma. If your facility is going to use siderails at all, then half-siderails are recommended. They prevent residents from rolling out of bed while allowing them to get up freely.

Several alternatives to bedrails have fewer negative consequences than those just discussed. Adjusting the height of the bed to ensure that a resident's feet can reach the ground when he or she is getting up is a good start. Consider buying beds that can be adjusted lower than the standard hospital bed height of 24 inches. In some cases, removing bed wheels is another possibility, but this must be approved by the local fire marshal. Beds are available with a mattress height of 12 inches at the lowest setting. Some facilities have begun to use platform beds on which the mattress is located only a few inches off the floor. Although this bed minimizes the risk of injury when a resident falls out of bed, staff find it awkward when they need to provide personal care. These beds should not be used for ambulatory residents, because a low bed can also restrain a resident from transferring independently. Another possibility is to place pads or foam mattresses around the bed of a nonambulatory resident.

If he or she falls out of bed, the pads or mattresses will help break the fall. This system is not recommended for ambulatory residents, who may slip and fall on these pads.

Communication Devices

Some alternatives to mechanical bed restraints include call bell systems and bed alarm systems (BASs). One problem with call bell systems is that residents with dementia may not understand how and when to use them. Therefore, a BAS that enables staff to know when a person is getting out of bed may be more useful. This type of system sounds an alarm at the nursing station when the resident leaves the bed but not when the person rolls over during sleep. The purpose of bed alarms is to alert staff to come quickly to the aid of a resident who needs assistance in getting to the bathroom or who should not walk unattended.

Several types of BASs are available (see "Where to Find Products"). Some versions attach to the bed and the resident. A sensor unit is mounted on the headboard and a garment clip is worn on the resident's nightclothes. When the resident gets up from the bed, the garment clip disengages from the sensor unit and activates the alarm. Another form of BAS consists of a small plastic unit that is attached to the resident's upper leg with a fabric band. When the person stands up, placing the sensor in a vertical position, the alarm is activated. Some alarms systems are attached directly to the bed in the form of pressure-sensitive pads that slip underneath the sheets or the mattress. When the person sits up, the motion activates the alarm. A pressure-sensitive carpet mat is another option.

The choice of a BAS is based on the individual attributes of the resident. Some residents with dementia may become agitated by the unfamiliar garment clip or leg device and remove it, thereby inactivating the system. Pressure-sensitive bed pads are likely to be a better alternative for these residents. Specific characteristics of the resident, such as body weight and sleep patterns, also play a role in choosing an effective system. One problem with devices that are not attached to the resident is that, by the time the alarm is activated, the resident is already out of bed. Staff do not have as much time to respond to the resident's bedroom. Another issue is that the less expensive systems have alarms that ring within 1 foot of the bed. This noise may be a source of agitation and confusion for the resident as well as others. When a resident continually sets off the alarm by accident, this leads to frustration.

Even though there may be an initial investment in implementing a BAS, the system can be well worth the cost. It may save money and staff time by reducing the frequency at which staff must do night checks. If the system works properly and reduces bed falls, then the savings from these costs alone makes the investment in the system pay off quickly. Although these devices are not entirely noninstitutional, they are far less invasive than mechanical bed restraints. To date, no studies have shown adverse effects from using BASs, and families prefer them for relatives because they offer more dignity than traditional bed restraints.

WHERE TO FIND PRODUCTS

Mobility Devices

The following companies carry a variety of walkers, wheelchairs, and other devices for helping residents remain mobile:

AbilityOne Corporation
4 Sammons Court
Bolingbrook, IL 60440
(800) 323-5547
www.sammonspreston.com

AliMed, Inc.
297 High Street
Dedham, MA 02026
(800) 225-2610
www.alimed.com

McKessonHBOC Medical Group
Extended Care Division (formerly Red Line HealthCare)
8121 10th Avenue North
Golden Valley, MN 55427
(800) 328-8111
www.redline.com

Merry Walker Corporation
11475 Commercial Avenue, Suite 9
Richmond, IL 60071
(815) 678-3388
www.merrywalker.com

Skil-Care
29 Wells Avenue
Yonkers, NY 10701
(800) 431-2972

Bed Alarm Systems

FallCare
c/o LabMARK Safety Systems
(530) 894-2520
e-mail: inform@fallcare.com

Guardian Electronics, Inc.
1001 W. Glen Oaks Lane, Suite 201
Mequon, WI 53092
(262) 241-4850
e-mail: sales@guardianbednet.com

RN+
4760 Walnut Street, Suite 105
Boulder, CO 80301
(800) 727-1868
www.rnplus.com

Lighting

ADA–Compliant Wall Sconces

SPI Lighting Inc.
10400 North Enterprise Drive
Mequon, WI 53092
(414) 242-1420
www.spilighting.com
Their Phaces wall sconces meet ADA's 4-inch clearance standard and
come with a variety of lighting options.

Lighting Consultants

Eunice Noell-Waggoner
Center for Design for an Aging Society
6200 S.W. Virginia Avenue, Suite 210
Portland, OR 97201
(503) 246-8231
Noell-Waggoner is an expert in the field of lighting for aging people.

Illuminating Engineering Society of North America
120 Wall Street, Floor 17
New York, NY 10005
(212) 248-5000
www.iesna.org
Lighting and the Visual Environment for Senior Living (1998)

Lighthouse International
111 East 59th Street
New York, NY 10022-1202
(800) 829-0500
www.lighthouse.org
Offers a variety of solutions and products for individuals with visual impairment

Flooring

Carpeting

Bonar Floors
365 Walt Sanders Memorial Drive
Newnan, GA 30265
(770) 252-4890
www.bonarfloors.com

Collins & Aikman Floorcoverings, Inc.
311 Smith Industrial Boulevard
Dalton, GA 30722-1447
(800) 248-2878
www.powerbond.com

Interface Flooring System, Inc.
Post Office Box 1503
LaGrange, GA 30241
(800) 336-0225
www.interfaceinc.com

Lees Commercial Carpets
3330 West Friendly Avenue
Post Office Box 26027
Greensboro, NC 27410
(800) 523-5647

Lowes Carpet Corporation
160 Duvall Road
Chatsworth, GA 30705
(800) 333-2468

Nonglare Resilient Flooring

Mannington Mills, Inc.
Post Office Box 30
Salem, NJ 08079
(800) 356-6787
www.mannington.com
Their Custom Spec II sheet vinyl line has a heavier sealer coat that does not require shiny polish. Colors and patterns have low contrast, and two patterns imitate a hardwood floor. Costs are only slightly higher than those of standard vinyl.

TOLI International
55 Mall Drive
Commack, NY 11725
(800) 446-5476
www.toli.com
Vinyl sheets and vinyl tile that are extremely durable and a variety look like hardwood floors. These products also have less sheen compared with other vinyl. Their Spectrafloors line is a textured product that, when left unpolished, diffuses glare. Costs are higher than for standard vinyl flooring, but the product is considered more durable.

Slip-Resistant Floors

Altro Floors
6390 Kestrel Road
Missassauga, Ontario L5T 1Z3, Canada
(800) 565-4658
www.Altrofloors.com
Manufactures Altro safety flooring, a slip-resistant sheet vinyl

Slip Tech
1111 La Mesa Avenue
Spring Valley, CA 91977
(800) 667-5470
Surface treatment for ceramic, tile, and concrete flooring to make it slip-resistant

Carpet-to-Tile Transitions

Johnsonite
16910 Munn Road
Chagrin Falls, OH 44023
(800) 899-8916
www.johnsonite.com

Communication Devices

Fidelity TeleAlarm LLC
2501 Kutztown Road
Reading, PA 19605-2961
(800) 483-0888
www.fidelitytelealarm.com
NurseCall, VoiceResponse, and Locate 1 with optional WanderCall wireless call systems

Hitec Communications
8160 Madison Avenue
Burr Ridge, IL 60521
(804) 288-6100
www.hitec.com
Integrated phone, call bell, and door monitoring system

Instantel Inc.
808 Commerce Park Drive
Ogdensburg, NY 13669
(800) 267-9111
www.instantel.com
WatchMate, a resident wanderer monitor system that has a silent paging option and can be connected to a computer program to log resident patterns

JTECH Communications, Inc.
6413 Congress Avenue
Suite 150
Boca Raton, FL 33487
(800) 321-6221
www.jtech.com
PeopleAlert Messaging System, a silent nurses' call system

Quiet Vacuum Cleaners

Newport Equipment Co., Inc.
24857 Broadway Avenue
Bedford, OH 44146
(440) 439-2224
Distributor of the NVQ 402 vacuum, a tank vacuum for institutional use made by North American Cleaning Equipment. This vacuum is rated at 50 dB at the location of the operator, which is well below the sound level of normal conversation.

Windsor Industries Inc.
1351 West Standford Avenue
Englewood, CO 80110
(800) 444-7654
www.windsorind.com
The Windsor Sensor is an upright vacuum cleaner for institutional use. This vacuum is rated at 69 dB at the location of the operator, which is the sound level of normal conversation. At 10 feet away, the sound level of the vacuum drops to 62 dB.

♦ ♦ ♦

A summary sheet follows, which condenses the chapter text into a quick overview. The authors have also provided an area for you to make your own notes about your own staff and facility. Managerial staff may wish to use the summary sheets as handouts to accompany direct care staff training, or to post them by the time clock or nurses' station or include them in staff's pay envelopes.

MOBILITY SUMMARY SHEET

1. Loss of mobility may affect function, autonomy, and psychological and physiological (musculoskeletal, neurological, cardiovascular, sensory) well-being.

2. Falls are a major source of disability in older adults. They result from both physiological changes and environmental factors. Falls have been related to moving to a new (and unfamiliar) living environment, mobility impairment, time of day, and low staff-to-resident ratios.

3. People with dementia are at a greater risk of falling than are people without dementia, they may experience balance and gait problems, and they may suffer from apraxia (difficulty with movement due to problems in processing motor skill information).

4. Many negative physical and emotional effects are associated with physical and chemical restraints. The use of physical restraints can significantly affect staff–resident relationships. Greater staff time is required to provide appropriate care to a large number of restrained residents.

What Staff Can Do

1. Monitor new residents closely, place residents who are at high risk of falls in rooms closer to staff work areas, stagger shift changes, and track near falls.

2. Encourage exercise programs as determined by the care team/resident because physical conditioning can help prevent falls and limit fall injuries. Exercise can be formal or part of ADLs. Sports or dancing can be fun/familiar ways to promote exercise. Monitor physical condition closely during exercise, especially in warm weather.

3. Resist the use of restraints. Alternatives include exercise to provide physical conditioning and social contact as well as reduce wandering, depression, aggression, and sleep disturbances; and rehabilitation, which requires taking special approaches with people with dementia, including short sessions centered on skills that they value.

4. Help residents to maintain continuity with past interests/activities when their mobility is significantly impaired. Focus on possibilities rather than limitations. Encourage friends to visit/find thoughtful things to do with residents.

5. Make mobility aids attractive/useful and treat them as "tools for living."

6. Support residents involved in rehabilitation programs by noticing/encouraging successes, writing notes/doing small extra services, helping them to walk or exercise.

7. Break ADLs into manageable parts; ensure that tired resident are not pushed to do more than they are able.

8. Plan rehabilitation programs that fit individual resident interests and needs.

9. Make sure therapy does not interfere with favorite or important activities or routines.

What the Environment Can Do

1. Provide high levels of even lighting, replace burned-out light bulbs immediately, and minimize glare.
2. Ensure that floor surfaces are level, and minimize color contrasts and patterns in flooring.
3. Keep hallways clear of clutter, and keep handrails clear.
4. Ensure that all furniture is stable in case residents use it to maintain their balance.

YOUR NOTES

4

Continence

Incontinent is defined as "unrestrained" or "unable to hold"; however, it is most often used to refer to the inability to control bowel and bladder movements. A number of factors increase the occurrence of incontinence as a part of normal aging. Dementia can further compound these factors. Also, issues that are related to relocation to a new living environment can increase incontinence. It is important to look at the causes of incontinence to find ways to help residents maintain continence. It is equally, if not more, important to address the feelings and needs of residents who have trouble maintaining continence.

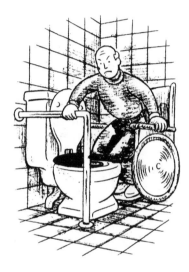

INCONTINENCE AS A PART OF NORMAL AGING

People are more likely to experience incontinence as they age. A number of physiological factors contribute to this problem. Some people experience *stress incontinence,* the involuntary loss of urine when they laugh, sneeze, or cough. Others may experience *urge incontinence,* the strong urge to urinate (void) but they are not able to make it to the bathroom in time. These are two of the more common forms of incontinence, and some people experience both. Other physiological causes relate to changes in the prostate or bladder, urinary tract infections, psychological disorders, and stool impaction. Some medications can also contribute to incontinence. In particular, sedatives, tranquilizers, and hypnotics can reduce a person's sensitivity to his or her body's sensations, including the urge to void.

Incontinence Compounded by Dementia

Elderly people with dementia may experience any of the above physiological factors related to incontinence, but these factors are compounded by their dementia. For instance, they may not recognize early urges to urinate and respond to them. When the urges become stronger, they may not remember the location of the bathroom or may not find it in time. The fact that people with dementia often lose the ability to plan ahead can increase their likelihood of being incontinent. Someone without cognitive impairment frequently thinks about going to the bathroom before he or she goes somewhere. For instance, residents without cognitive impairment may intentionally go to the bathroom before going to the dining room for dinner or the activity room for a movie, so that they do not need to interrupt what they are doing later. Residents with dementia may no longer be able to plan ahead in this way.

Living in a long-term care facility can have effects on continence as well. Residents with dementia may never become as familiar with the facility as they were with their own homes, and they may have continuous difficulty finding the bathrooms in the facility. Likewise, some facilities have toilets only in the bedrooms and tub rooms, and these may not be clearly identified (see "What the Environment Can Do" later in this chapter).

Immobility can cause incontinence as well. Residents who are unable to leave their beds, are restrained, or use gerichairs are more likely than residents who are mobile to become incontinent. When these residents need to urinate, they cannot get to the bathroom on their own and may not be able to communicate with staff before an accident occurs.

CHANGES IN A RESIDENT'S CONTINENCE

When a resident begins to have episodes of incontinence, or an increase in the frequency of them, it is important to request a medical examination. As mentioned in the beginning of this section, a number of physiological factors can contribute to incontinence. Many of these factors, especially urinary tract infections, can and must be treated.

Once physiological factors have been ruled out or treated, other issues that could cause incontinence must be explored for each resident. A number of programmatic strategies can be employed for reducing incontinence and reducing resident embarrassment when toileting assistance is needed. In addition, a number of environmental modifications can make finding bath-

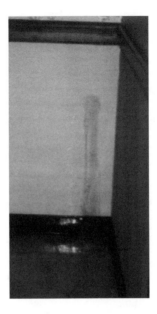

Figure 4.1. When residents with cognitive impairment cannot find bathrooms or are not able to plan ahead, incontinence problems can result.

rooms easier for residents with dementia (Figure 4.1). These modifications are covered in the following two sections.

WHAT STAFF CAN DO

Interventions

Staff should be aware of both the physiological and environmental factors that can challenge the ability of residents with dementia to maintain continence. To the extent possible, staff should make alterations in the physical environment that allow ambulatory residents to continue to use the bathroom independently as much as possible. This may minimize their embarrassment of having to ask for, or receive, assistance with toileting. However, environmental interventions will not work for all residents. This section discusses some staff-based approaches for maintaining residents' continence and assisting with toileting that may be particularly effective.

Step-by-Step Cueing

Some residents may lose their sense of what to do when they get to the bathroom. This does not necessarily mean they need physical assistance. Step-by-step cueing helps residents maintain some personal control over the situation. Always allow residents to do as much by themselves as they can. Often, verbal cueing and hand gestures for each step are all that are needed. When a resident does not seem to understand one of the steps, staff may need to physically assist him or her to complete that step, but they should then go back to verbal cueing for the next step. You can write out a list of steps for toileting to share with direct care staff. Examples of specific steps in the process include unzipping and/or pulling down pants, sitting on toilet, voiding or having a bowel movement, tearing off toilet paper, and so on.

Using Sequencing Cards with Toileting

Given the verbal and language impairments of residents with dementia, some may not understand what staff are trying to do when assisting them with toileting. Consider developing a set of sequencing cards with illustrations that show the various steps of toileting (see "Where to Find Products" for sources). The first card might show a resident in his or her clothes approaching a toilet. The second card might show a resident unbuttoning or pulling his or her clothes down. The third card could show a resident sitting on the toilet. The fourth card could show a resident reaching for the toilet paper. The fifth card could show a resident pulling up/fastening his or her clothing. The next few cards would show a resident going through the steps of washing and drying his or her hands. Additional information about sequencing cards can be found under "Sequence of Dressing" in Chapter 6 in this volume.

Scheduled/Preventive Toileting

Scheduled toileting often helps to reduce the frequency of incontinent episodes. Staff offers toileting assistance or cueing every 2–3 hours for all residents who have difficulty remaining continent. A more tailored approach to toileting is to develop individualized toileting schedules. To do this, staff need to spend time observing the patterns of residents who have trouble maintaining continence. Direct care staff should try to record each time they are aware of residents going to the bathroom or being incontinent for a few days. They can use the Behavior Tracking Form for monitoring toileting behaviors (see

Volume 3, Appendix A; an explanation of the behavior tracking process can be found in Chapter 1 of that volume). Once staff can predict when residents need to use the bathroom, individual toileting programs can be developed for each of them. Develop a schedule to have staff offer assistance or cueing shortly before they anticipate residents' needing to relieve themselves.

Fluid Consumption

Staff sometimes may make the mistake of reducing the fluid intake of residents who are prone to incontinence. This practice does not reduce incontinence and actually can result in an increase in its occurrence. Drinking less than the recommended 6 cups of fluid daily results in urine becoming highly concentrated, which irritates the bladder and can result in increased incontinence. Observing patterns of liquid consumption, however, may help to predict residents' need to void.

Reducing Embarrassment When Assistance Is Needed

Staff must remember that assisting residents with toileting is more than simply another task. Staff must consider residents' feelings about their own continence, or lack thereof, and any toileting assistance that they need. Episodes of incontinence can be embarrassing to people. Even a person with dementia likely feels a loss of self-control and shame when incontinent. Likewise, going to the bathroom is a private act, and being accompanied to the bathroom is discomforting for most people. In addition to the embarrassment and general unease felt by residents generally, residents with dementia may not understand what is being asked of them.

Understandably, dealing with episodes of urine and bowel incontinence are one of the staff's least desirable, though necessary, tasks. Helping a resident after he or she has been incontinent can be an unpleasant experience, as can assisting a combative resident with toileting. In addition, staff may feel uncomfortable because they know that the resident is embarrassed and uncomfortable about being approached by them about toileting or changing clothes. These issues can cause staff to postpone this kind of care. Talk to staff in facilities with a scheduled toileting program about their feelings concerning helping residents try to maintain continence. Share with them the approaches that can make this more comfortable for all involved.

Most people are more comfortable with staff members of the same gender when it comes to personal care such as toileting. When a resident needs assistance in the bathroom or needs to be changed after an episode of incontinence, ask a staff member of the same gender, with whom the resident is comfortable, to assist. When approaching residents about assistance with toileting, be as discrete as possible and speak into their ear. Even when residents need help in the bathroom, it is important to provide as much privacy as possible. For residents who need step-by-step cueing, staff can step back a bit or turn their back while they are helping residents in the bathroom. After providing any help needed with clothing and seating, staff can step outside the bathroom while the resident completes toileting, a time when residents likely appreciate privacy the most. When the resident is done, the staff member can return and provide any assistance that is necessary.

WHAT THE ENVIRONMENT CAN DO

The process of going to the bathroom independently requires several steps. Residents first must be able to find the bathroom, which means placing clearly visible cues on the outside of the bathroom door as well as inside the bathroom. Second, they must be able to find the toilet within the bathroom, which can be surprisingly challenging. Finally, they must be able to manage removing clothing and transferring to the toilet.

Finding the Bathroom

Increasing the visibility of doors to common bathrooms may help residents find these rooms quickly and may help staff direct residents to the toilet because they can refer to a distinguishing feature. Some facilities paint bathroom doors a bright color that contrasts with that of the wall. Common bathrooms also should have large, highly visible signs with printed words that are easy to read or with simple, clear graphics (Figure 4.2). Signs on the floor (see "Where to Find Products") or fabric canopies mounted over the door are other strategies that can be used to call attention to these rooms (Namazi & Johnson, 1991b). Over-the-door canopies can be less institutional looking than using large signs (Figure 4.3). Canopies can be made from window valances if the bathroom door opens into the room. Stuff the valance with tissue paper to make it stand out more. Both features are uncommon enough that they will likely grab residents' attention. The same strategies can be used for bathrooms that are located adjacent to residents' rooms.

Finding the Toilet

Once a resident finds a bathroom, he or she must be able to easily find the toilet in the room. This may be difficult for a person with poor vision or im-

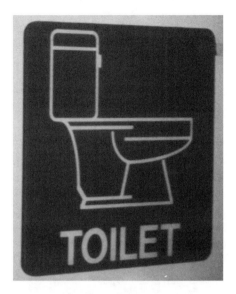

Figure 4.2.   Large, simple signs can be
used to identify the location of toilets.

paired cognitive abilities. Increasing the visibility of toilets can be effective in
maintaining continence. For these residents, a toilet that is out of sight may
never be found. Research in one facility that used a curtain in place of a bathroom door found that toilets hidden by drawn curtains were used 37 times in
45 hours of observation. When the curtains were pulled back so that the toilet was visible, the toilets were used 285 times in 45 hours (Namazi & Johnson,
1991a). Look for ways to increase visibility if the toilets in residents' bedrooms
are not easily visible from their bed. Try removing the bathroom door and replacing it with a curtain. Each facility should decide whether privacy or maintaining continence is more important when trying these interventions. If
bathroom doors can be left open at night, help residents to find the toilet by
installing a night-light in the bathroom.

When the floor, toilet fixtures, and walls are the same color, it may be
difficult for residents with poor vision to see the toilet. Consider painting
bathroom walls a different color so that the fixtures stand out. If this is not
possible, try changing the color of the toilet seat so it has a more prominent
appearance. Before investing in new seats, place a strip of colored tape
around the edge of the seats to determine whether this change is effective.
Changing the color of the toilet seat is also more cost effective than changing
the color of the bathroom floor. Facilities planning to remodel or alter bathroom walls or floors should keep the idea of color contrast in mind.

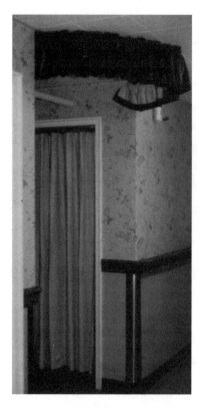

Figure 4.3. Fabric canopies mounted over the bathroom door can help residents find the toilet.

Some residents void in a sink or wastebasket. These episodes should be viewed as attempts to maintain continence—these residents really were trying to find the appropriate place to void, and these receptacles may have been more visible than the toilet. Consider either removing the wastebasket, placing it in a more discrete area (e.g., under the sink), or replacing it with one with a lid.

Transferring to and from the Toilet

The process of transferring to, sitting on, and using a toilet takes a degree of dexterity and balance. In many cases a resident may be able to perform this process independently without requiring staff assistance if the appropriate grab bar is in place (Figure 4.4). Older facilities may not have adequate grab bars, or may have placed them in inaccessible locations. Although ADA has encouraged the removal of these barriers, this legislation does not force a facility to modify every bathroom. Before installing new grab bars, a facility

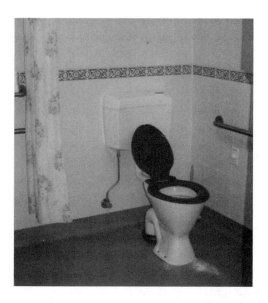

Figure 4.4. An example of an easily located and accessible toilet with a curtain and contrasting toilet seat and lid for better visibility and appropriately placed grab bar.

should refer to ADA and state guidelines regarding what is appropriate. ADA guidelines suggest that grab bars should be located behind and on at least one side of a toilet. The side grab bars should extend in front of the toilet so that they are easy to reach. The diameter of a grab bar should be between 1¼ and 1½ inches so that it can be gripped easily. Grab bars should be mounted on the wall 32–36 inches above the floor. Make sure that towel bars and other wall-mounted items can hold the weight of a resident, because they may be used for support along with grab bars when transferring.

ADA guidelines were not written with older adults or people with dementia in mind, so additional grab bars may be needed to customize a toilet for specific residents. For example, a resident may not be able to transfer to the toilet unless a vertical grab bar (mounted 40 inches above the floor and located 12 inches from the toilet) is provided. ADA guidelines also make it difficult for a two-person transfer to occur easily in bathrooms, which can pose a problem in a facility with people with physical impairments. Sometimes devices can be used that meet ADA–equivalent standards, such as a swing-down grab bar. Also, the toilet paper dispenser must be within easy reach and should not require a great deal of force to use.

It can be difficult to transfer a person easily from a wheelchair to a toilet in a small bathroom. New and remodeled bathrooms should accommodate a resident in a wheelchair and a caregiver comfortably. A clear floor space should be provided on at least one side of the toilet for easy transfer with staff assistance.

WHERE TO FIND PRODUCTS

Sequencing Cards

Imaginart
307 Arizona Street
Bisbee, AZ 85603
(800) 828-1376
e-mail: imaginart@aol.com
Pick 'n Stick communication products

Mayer-Johnson, Inc.
Post Office Box 1597
Solana Beach, CA 92075
(800) 588-4548
www.mayer-johnson.com
Manufacturer of Boardmaker and Board-Builder

Toilet Signs for the Floor

Consolidated Plastics
(800) 362-1000
Consolidated Plastics stencils logos onto floor mats. You can have the word *toilet* with an arrow stenciled on the mat. This mat can be used outside a common bathroom to cue residents that there is a toilet inside the room. Remember to make the background color match the color of the surrounding flooring so that residents do not avoid this area because they think it is a hole in the floor.

Colored Toilet Seats

Kohler Company
444 Highland Drive
Kohler, WI 53044
(800) 456-4537
www.kohlerco.com
Manufactures open-front colored toilet seats (also available by special order through your local home building supply warehouse)

Grab Bars

AbilityOne Corporation
4 Sammons Court
Bolingbrook, IL 60440
(800) 323-5547
www.sammonspreston.com

AliMed, Inc.
297 High Street
Dedham, MA 02026
(800) 225-2610
www.alimed.com

Anchor Architectural Products
3106 Pleasant View Drive
Manheim, PA 17545
(717) 314-6552

Bobrick
(518) 877-7444
Call for the name of your local representative.

SeaChrome Corporation
9819 Klingerman Street
South El Monte, CA 91733
(800) 955-2476
www.seachrome.com

Waterproof Fabrics

Fantagraph
1 Knollcrest Drive
Cincinnati, OH 45237
(800) 888-5000
www.fantagraph.com
Manufactures a broad range of waterproof fabrics in residential styles

♦ ♦ ♦

A summary sheet follows, which condenses the chapter text into a quick overview. The authors have also provided an area for you to make your own notes about your own staff and facility. Managerial staff may wish to use the summary sheets as handouts to accompany direct care staff training, or to post them by the time clock or nurses' station or include them in staff's pay envelopes.

CONTINENCE SUMMARY SHEET

1. Incontinence is the inability to control bladder or bowel movements.
2. Urinary incontinence may occur with laughing, coughing, or sneezing (stress incontinence), with feeling a sudden strong urge to go (urge incontinence), or with having illnesses or taking certain medications.
3. People with dementia may not recognize early urges to go, and they may have difficulty finding a toilet in time.
4. People with dementia have difficulty anticipating and planning for the future. They may fail to plan to toilet before a meal, car ride, or activity.
5. Immobility, restraints, and the fact that toilets can be difficult to find in long-term care settings also contribute to incontinence.
6. A thorough medical assessment is important to determine whether incontinence is caused by a medical problem or illness.

What Staff Can Do

1. Make sure bathrooms can be easily used independently.
2. Provide step-by-step cueing or use picture cue cards.
3. Maintain individual toilet schedules, and encourage regular fluid consumption.
4. Reduce embarrassment by involving same-sex caregivers and promoting privacy.

What the Environment Can Do

1. Make toilet doorway easy to spot with contrasting paint or canopy, and provide good signage at appropriate levels.
2. Make toilets easily visible with good lighting, open doors, and contrast among toilet/seat/walls/floor.
3. Remember that voiding in objects such as wastebaskets is an attempt to maintain continence. Make toilets more visible than wastebaskets or move wastebaskets to a shelf or a less obvious place.
4. Ensure safe transfers in toilet areas. Grab bars should be properly placed with adequate space for making wheelchair transfers.

YOUR NOTES

5

Eating

Food is much more than nutrition. For most people, eating is one of life's basic pleasures. It symbolizes daily nurturing and caring. Food is an important part of virtually all of life's celebrations—holidays, birthdays, weddings, and many other happy occasions. From childhood on, people often associate food with familiar events and fun activities. For instance, eating popcorn at the movies or a hot dog at the ballpark are experiences that many Americans have shared. Food also may evoke special memories, such as the smell of turkey at Thanksgiving, grilling hamburgers for a Fourth of July cookout, or baking and decorating Christmas cookies.

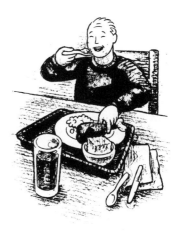

Many people have specific tastes and preferences when it comes to food. Some people only want to eat fresh fruits and vegetables, whereas others may find canned or frozen food perfectly acceptable. Typically, people have their own special ways of preparing various dishes. They may not enjoy these foods as much when they are cooked in other ways (e.g., a person who is used to homemade mashed potatoes may not enjoy instant potatoes). In some cultures, people are accustomed to having specific ethnic foods such as tortillas or rice offered with every meal. Without them, the food served may not seem like a meal.

Not all people want to eat the standard three meals per day. Some people regularly eat lots of small snacks throughout the day instead of two or three large meals. Some people do not like to eat breakfast at all, others prefer just coffee and toast, whereas still others enjoy eating a full breakfast such as pancakes and sausages. At lunchtime, some people may view a bowl of soup and a piece of bread as a meal, whereas for others that may be a first course. Certain people are used to raiding the refrigerator around 9:00–10:00 P.M. for a snack, whereas others would never dream of eating anything after dinnertime.

People have many different ideas about food. These ideas often develop in childhood and may last a lifetime or continue to evolve as a person ages. Knowing an individual's food tastes and preferences makes it much easier to prepare food that he or she will like and want to eat.

HOW EATING CHANGES WITH AGE

Social Issues

At every stage of life, favorite foods can be a source of comfort and happiness. One author said that eating is a "barometer of emotional as well as physical well being" (Hellen, 1990). Good food smells may remind residents of long-term care facilities of home, family, and happy times. Smells such as freshly baked homemade bread or brewed coffee are especially comforting when residents are stressed, ill, or depressed. It is not surprising that, for many residents, mealtimes are highlights of the day. Yet, there are many psychological reasons why residents may not want to eat. Older people who lived alone prior to moving into a facility may be used to eating sandwiches or other easy-to-prepare foods. The larger meals served in a facility may seem overwhelming to them. Poor health and depression frequently diminish the appetites of older people as well.

Eating may become less pleasurable for older adults when they cannot see, smell, or taste well or hear conversations at the table. It also may be embarrassing if they have trouble handling utensils and notice others watching them. Furthermore, residents with early-stage dementia who recognize their losses may feel depressed and not want to eat. Heightened anxiety relating to increasing confusion, forgetfulness, and difficulties in navigating the environment also may cause a loss of appetite. Sometimes residents may believe that they want to "give up and die," and therefore cease to eat.

Physical Issues

Many physical conditions related to aging also can cause eating difficulties. Treating physical symptoms promptly is important because eating well helps older people to maintain overall good health, prevent skin breakdown, decrease constipation, and boost the immune system. Always obtain a medical evaluation to determine whether a specific resident's eating problems are due to physiological conditions. Problems relating to the mouth, throat, hands, and digestive system may have a great impact on eating. Because there are many good clinical resources available focusing on these specific issues, we will not spend much time on them. Instead, the following text briefly highlights how several of these factors can contribute to the eating difficulties that older people experience.

Multiple sensory losses that occur with aging make it harder to eat and limit the pleasure derived from food (see Volume 1 for more information). Low vision affects the ability of older people to see what they are eating and to locate the food on their plates or the appropriate utensils on the table. Some residents may also have trouble distinguishing between different foods on their plates, especially when the foods are similar in color. Others may have trouble judging where the edges of the plate are and may be more likely to spill food. Poor hearing has an impact on the ability to enjoy conversation and participate in the social aspects of eating. Diminished senses of smell and taste because of certain medications and normal aging greatly limit the pleasure of eating. Even a reduced tactile sense makes it hard to identify various foods and utensils on the table.

Many older adults also experience problems with mouth pain that may worsen eating problems (Figure 5.1). For instance, they may experience difficulties in eating comfortably when they have problems such as sores in the mouth, dry mouth, missing or no teeth, or ill-fitting dentures. In general,

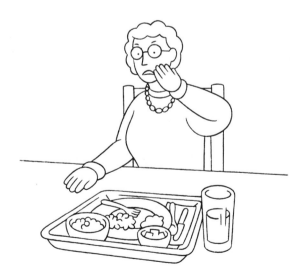

Figure 5.1.   Some residents may experience difficulty eating because of mouth pain.

mouth pain is a treatable problem that should be evaluated by medical staff so that they can identify appropriate solutions to minimize eating difficulties.

Problems such as tremor, rigidity, and poor coordination may cause eating to be exceedingly frustrating for residents. Serving finger foods that can be picked up easily may make a major difference for these residents (Zgola & Bordillon, 2001). Physical and occupational therapists can recommend assistive devices to help older people with these problems eat more independently. (For specific suggestions about available assistive devices, refer to "Where to Find Products" at the end of the chapter.)

Many types of gastrointestinal problems cause older people to experience pain or discomfort from eating. Often, knowing in advance that such problems are likely to occur may affect their desire to eat. Another common problem is that older adults may become fearful that they will need to use the bathroom immediately after eating and will not be able to get there in time. Seating these residents closest to the dining room door or their knowing that staff will assist them quickly when they have urgent needs can help reduce these worries.

HOW DEMENTIA AFFECTS THE EXPERIENCE OF EATING

Residents with dementia not only experience age-related problems but they also commonly experience eating difficulties that result from their cognitive impairments. These residents may lose their understanding of the body's physical need for nourishment. Over time, they may no longer understand the purpose of eating or may not even recognize food. Even if they can identify the food, they may have forgotten the social skills of dining, such as the use of a fork or a napkin.

Occasionally, food may be associated with negative life experiences (e.g., being violently ill after eating a particular food). Even for residents with late-stage dementia, seeing, smelling, or eating certain foods may trigger memories that produce strong emotional reactions. These reactions may occur even in people who are otherwise uncommunicative. In addition, some older adults have experienced certain events that influence their overall attitudes about the handling of food. For example, people who lacked adequate food during the Depression or World War II may respond now by hoarding food whenever it is presented to them. They may overeat not from hunger but from a fear that they will not receive food later.

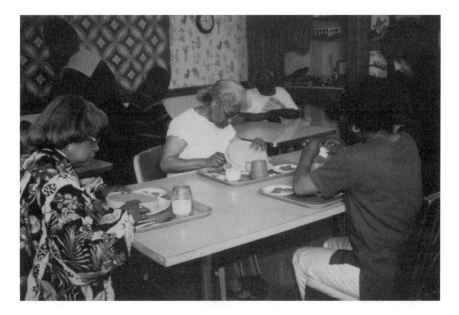

Figure 5.2. Residents with dementia may have trouble concentrating on eating if the dining room atmosphere is overstimulating.

Memory Problems

In early-stage dementia, recent memory and concentration are affected, and residents may have trouble remembering the times and location of meals. They may be embarrassed that they cannot remember where the dining room is and feel badly if they have to ask repeatedly for help in finding it. If the facility or unit has a multipurpose room that is used for meals rather than a dedicated dining room, then this may add to their confusion. Ways to help residents with dementia in finding the dining room are discussed in "What the Environment Can Do."

Beyond finding the dining room, residents with dementia may have trouble concentrating on eating if the dining room environment overstimulates them (Figure 5.2). They may be distracted easily by a number of factors, including the number of items on the table (e.g., condiments, silverware, napkins), the number of people in the room, and the noise level. Ways to make the dining experience less stimulating for these residents are discussed in "What Staff Can Do" and "What the Environment Can Do."

When residents with dementia start to experience increased memory loss, they not only may forget where meals are served and have trouble concentrating on eating but also forget when they last ate. Consequently, they may forget that they have just eaten a meal and ask for more food. Some professionals have suggested that such overeating in the initial stages of dementia is not a major problem because it cushions the resident against future weight loss (Hall, 1994; Hellen, 1990). Despite not always perceiving hunger or thirst, people with dementia continue to need to consume sufficient calories and drink enough fluids, especially when they are physically active (e.g., wanderers). People with dementia are also less likely than people without dementia to notice that they are thirsty and become dehydrated. Even if they do notice their thirst, many of these residents may not able to act on it and drink when they need to. Therefore, some residents with dementia may not be drinking the minimum of 6 cups (1.5 liters) of fluid per day that are needed for adequate hydration. This inadequate intake is a serious issue, especially because many medications commonly taken by residents may cause dehydration.

Problems with Chewing and Swallowing

As the dementing illness progresses further, residents may forget the basic processes of eating, such as chewing and swallowing. *Dysphagia* is the impaired ability to chew and swallow. This problem is one of the main reasons for malnutrition in people with dementia and can be life threatening. Dysphagia can cause a person to *aspirate,* or accidentally inhale particles of food while attempting to swallow. When these food particles become lodged in the lungs,

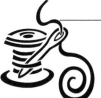

Eating on the Run

Staff should fit the environment around residents' needs rather than the other way around. Wanderers and excessive walkers have special eating problems because of the limited time that they spend sitting and the amount of energy they expend in continuous physical activity. For these residents, the eating environment may need to extend beyond the dining room. Think of ways to provide nutritional supplements (e.g., finger foods, snacks on the run) that address their nutritional needs. Hall (1994) suggested making waist pouches that enable residents to carry finger foods, including high-calorie snacks, with them at all times. If you have a problem with wanderers hiding finger foods as they walk around the unit, then offer them single bite-size pieces as they make their way around.

swelling can occur, producing pneumonia and other pulmonary infections. Aspiration is one of the primary causes of death in people with dementia (Hall, 1994).

Staff must investigate why residents are experiencing difficulties with chewing and swallowing. Mechanical problems such as an obstruction of the esophagus may be causing pain. In some cases, overmedicating (e.g., with sedatives) may contribute to chewing and swallowing difficulties. Later in the course of dementia, residents may forget the process of chewing and may be able to eat foods only when their textures have been altered to ease swallowing.

When Residents Are No Longer Able to Eat

People with late-stage dementia may completely lose the ability to eat and drink. This process occurs gradually as residents first lose the ability to use utensils and later become unable to remember basic functions such as chewing and swallowing. These residents commonly experience significant weight loss, are frequently immobile, and return to infantile grasping and sucking reflexes. These changes may necessitate both substantial diet modification and complete staff assistance with feeding.

At this point, choices must be made among different feeding strategies, including hand feeding, a nasogastric tube, or a permanent gastrostomy tube. These are difficult decisions for families to make for their loved ones. Staff can counsel families who are faced with making a decision about a feeding strategy. Ideally, these issues should be discussed before the situation reaches a crisis point.

Staff should take a palliative approach and maintain oral feeding as long as possible. Although artificial feeding methods may have medical advantages in preventing further weight loss, their impact on the residents' quality of life must be considered seriously. Using a feeding tube completely removes the sensory experience of eating because residents neither taste the food nor have human contact with staff. It also means that often residents "who might otherwise be ambulatory must be medically or pharmacologically confined to a bed or a gerichair to prevent them from removing the tube" (Volicer et al., 1989, p. 193). In cases in which a nasogastric tube is used as a temporary measure to ensure adequate nutrition while an eating problem is being diagnosed, have a strategy in place for removing the tube as soon as possible. For residents who must use a feeding tube permanently, it is important for staff to maintain at least the social aspects of eating, such as conversation and human touch.

WHAT STAFF CAN DO

Although good nutrition is clearly a goal in all long term-care facilities, it can be a significant challenge for residents with dementia. A team approach involving nursing staff, dietitians, occupational therapists, and speech-language pathologists addresses eating difficulties most effectively. A multidisciplinary team can brainstorm ways to minimize excess disability and enhance residents' abilities to eat independently.

Reasons that Residents May Reject Food

Even when residents with dementia experience serious difficulties with eating, staff must remember that they are people with feelings and should treat them with respect and support them. When residents' abilities are supported, they are more content, less frustrated, and better able to maintain their overall food consumption. A way to treat residents with respect is for staff to not perceive mealtimes as simply a chore to be handled three times per day. Rather, meals should be viewed as social opportunities and an important activity for staff and residents. Meals provide a chance for older adults to enjoy companionship while eating. Conversation is one of the major aspects of a meal in any setting, especially a group setting. Whenever possible, staff should try to promote dining room conversation by grouping residents for social reasons such as common interests and compatible personalities, rather than exclusively based on functional ability. Unhappiness with dining companions can significantly reduce residents' appetites and consequently their food intake.

Residents also may not want to eat because they miss their familiar routines from home (Figure 5.3). Staff should validate residents' lifelong eating patterns. Try to learn about each resident's eating habits from the person or from family members and retain those rituals (e.g., two cups of black coffee in the morning, a mug of hot milk at bedtime). This type of subtle cueing may help increase residents' orientation to time of day. Furthermore, using familiar signals (e.g., inviting a resident to wash his or her hands before dinner) may help a resident with dementia to remember that this routine is associated with mealtimes. Try to maintain the regular courses that people eat during a meal. Do not serve all of the food at one time, but rather offer courses sequentially, one at a time (e.g., serve the entrée before dessert).

Because the tastes of people with dementia may change over time, even residents who have loved certain foods throughout their lives may suddenly develop aversions to them. Be flexible in terms of what is offered, and keep

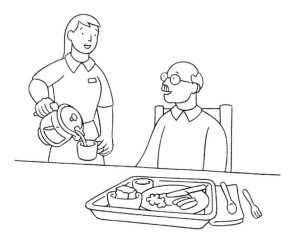

Figure 5.3.   It is important to preserve familiar routines for residents, such as drinking a cup of coffee before breakfast.

trying new foods, even with picky eaters. Occasionally, a new food can be introduced to determine whether people like it. If certain residents refuse particular foods, then offer other items from the complete meal.

Identifying foods that residents still enjoy definitely can help boost their total consumption. Ostasz (1986) suggested that, if certain residents love desserts, then extra milk can be mixed into puddings or added like a glaze over a piece of cake to make these dishes both more nutritious and easier to swallow. Sometimes, combining fruit in gelatin, cottage cheese, or cereal varies the texture and makes these foods more desirable to residents than when they are offered individually. Because many residents with dementia may have an age-related diminishment in their sense of taste, they may prefer foods with stronger flavors (e.g., heavily sweetened lemonade, salty foods). Food acceptance or rejection is largely based on a combination of how the food looks, smells, and tastes. Close observation of residents with eating problems will provide clues to their preferences regarding consistency, temperature, and features of food (e.g., smooth, cold, crunchy).

Staff awareness of the eating preferences of specific residents will help them to interpret their signals more accurately. For example, if a particular food served causes an extreme or catastrophic reaction in a resident, investigate whether there is an explanation for this behavior that is related to his or her personal history. Make sure that this reaction is documented so that the food is not served to the resident again. Knowing the individual dining patterns of specific residents, such as whether they prefer to socialize or limit conversation at meals, or whether they like to have a second cup of coffee, can make meals more pleasurable for everyone. Consistent staffing can facilitate personalized care for residents and may minimize eating problems in some individuals.

Hellen (1990) noted that some residents with dementia are reluctant to eat when they believe that family members are coming to visit and they want to wait to eat the meal with them. This issue must be handled sensitively to validate these residents' feelings and not upset them prior to the meal, which may affect their ability to eat. Hellen suggested placing an extra chair next to these residents to indicate that a place has been saved for their loved ones.

Similarly, Hellen suggests that some residents with dementia may be reluctant to accept food when they believe that they have not paid for it. Receiving a tray may lead them to believe that they are in a restaurant or a cafeteria, where they are supposed to pay for the food served. Some facilities have worked around this problem by giving the residents meal tickets that are punched or telling them that meals are covered by insurance or Medicare. Some residents, however, may not believe that the meal is either free or has been prepaid. Either serving food without trays or removing food from trays at the table may help in resolving this problem (Hellen, 1990).

It is important for staff to realize that social norms vary regarding basic issues such as how one behaves at the table, what is considered appropriate to leave on your plate, and table manners. Knowing a resident's social norms and values can help staff to develop an appropriate strategy to encourage the resident to eat. The following is a good example (Moody, 1992):

Miss W., an 87 year old woman, had been refusing to go down to the dining room and eat meals for a period of several weeks. Nursing staff had charted a significant weight loss and were starting to discuss the issue of compulsory feeding for her. At this time, a young social worker who had a good relationship with Miss W. invited her "out to lunch." Miss W. accepted, saying that she had never been one to turn down an invitation to lunch. So they went and dined at a separate table in the dining room. This lunch invitation was what it took to get Miss W. to return to eating in the dining room. After this, she began to regularly attend meals in the dining room and eventually regained her strength. Occasionally, the social worker continued to come by and invite her to lunch. (pp. 141–142)

This lovely example shows how using the resident's lifelong perception of herself as a gracious lady who never turned down a formal invitation helped to encourage her to return to eating in the dining room. In this case, it proved to be a more dignified alternative to the clinical interventions that were being proposed for handling her eating problems.

Beyond psychological factors, staff also should be trained to understand how eating abilities change over the course of dementia. It is important to recognize that residents with dementia are not just being stubborn or willful when they do not eat. Eating problems are not necessarily the fault of either the residents or the staff but part of the progression of dementia. However, staff may feel pressured because state inspectors often closely monitor residents' weight loss. Consequently, if residents do not regularly eat 75%–80% of meals, then staff may be afraid that they will be blamed for poor care. The goal should not be to assign blame but instead to brainstorm ways to prevent further weight loss. One way to do this is to create a more therapeutic setting for dining.

Creating a Therapeutic Setting for Dining

Many aspects are involved in creating a therapeutic setting for dining. The focus here is on what staff can do; "What the Environment Can Do" examines ways to modify the dining room. Some of the most therapeutic actions that staff can take are to create a pleasant atmosphere in which to dine, minimize distractions, and provide appropriate cues for residents (Zgola & Bordillon, 2001). Noise and distractions can be minimized by eliminating the use of the public address system in the dining area and turning off televisions and loud music. Staff should not yell or talk loudly to one another because this may distract residents with dementia from concentrating on eating. The playing of soft, calming music during meals is controversial. Some experts in the field of dementia contend that even playing soft classical music can be distracting for some residents. Conversely, some research has suggested that quiet music can play a positive role in reducing incidents of agitated behavior, including those occurring at mealtimes. Denney (1997) provided a good literature review summarizing studies conducted on this topic.

Ensuring good nutritional intake while preserving the functional independence of residents with dementia can be time consuming. People with dementia may require significantly more time than other people to finish eating a meal. Too often, the conventional time frame allocated for meals does not permit residents with dementia to be active participants in the meal process. Yet, if the setting is designed to be therapeutic, then it is necessary to prioritize residents' abilities to eat independently over various bureaucratic and organizational time constraints.

Administrative Support

Facility administration must fully support staff in their efforts to make dining therapeutic. One good idea is to implement a mentoring program so that staff who are experienced in working with residents with eating problems can provide assistance to and support other staff. Mentors also can help brainstorm methods of coping with the particular eating difficulties of individual residents. Furthermore, mentors can work with family members and volunteers to train them in various aspects of assisting with eating, including proper positioning, rate of feeding, how to recognize the clinical signs of aspiration, and use of appropriate verbal and physical cues.

Not all changes to addressing residents' eating problems will take money or staff time to implement. For example, staff can improve the eating abilities of residents with dementia by doing simple things such as reminding residents to insert their dentures before meals. Another approach is to increase the number of finger foods served. One research study in an Alzheimer's care center with 54 residents specifically examined the effects of increasing the number of finger foods served (Soltesz & Dayton, 1995). The findings showed that increasing the number of finger foods did boost overall food consumption among these residents. Although most participants did not gain weight, they also did not lose weight, as commonly occurs in residents with Alzheimer's disease. More important, these authors noted that making a simple change such as increasing the number of finger foods served at this facility did not require staff to learn new skills or take extra staff time.

Using the 5 Ws to Analyze Eating Problems

Eating is both an activity and a process with stages that can be analyzed to understand what works and what does not work. Staff can use the 5 Ws to analyze eating problems. (The 5 Ws—who, what [e.g., what behavior], where, when, and why—are a part of the Behavior Tracking Process that is explained in Volume 3, Chapter 1.) Think about which residents are having eating difficulties and why these difficulties are occurring. What is being served, and what else is going on in the environment at mealtimes? Where does the resident sit in the dining area, and how does that location affect overall food consumption? Finally, when does the resident experience eating difficulties? Is it an ongoing problem or does it occur just at certain times of the day (e.g., breakfast)?

Once the 5 Ws have been used to identify and track the problem, staff can talk about how to provide appropriate assistance for different residents. When a specific resident's eating abilities are being discussed during a care

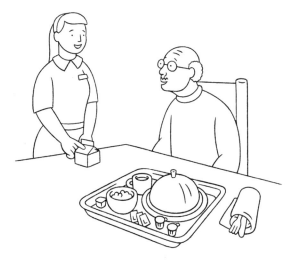

Figure 5.4. Staff may need to provide only minimal assistance for residents before they eat.

planning conference, for example, it is also useful to solicit input from the individuals most involved in providing direct care, such as the nursing assistants who often work with this resident. In addition, the Behavior Tracking Form (see Volume 3, Appendix A) may be used to monitor the effectiveness of various interventions in increasing specific residents' food consumption. The focus should be on not only those who need total assistance, but also other residents with dementia who could eat independently with a small amount of extra assistance or with modest changes in the meal service.

Providing Different Levels of Assistance

Residents who require minimal assistance may need help opening milk cartons or unwrapping utensils (Figure 5.4). They also may need occasional verbal cues to encourage them to eat. These residents may be able to concentrate better on the task at hand if their food is served one course at a time. Again, in general, finger foods are easier to eat than are foods requiring the use of utensils. Finger foods can be defined broadly to include soups in a mug and nutritious drinks as well as solid foods. In some cases, families may need to be educated about the benefits of finger foods and why they are being served more frequently to their loved ones than are other types of food.

Residents who require moderate assistance may be unable to chew the foods included in a regular diet without some modifications. Most of these residents still can swallow but may need to be reminded to do so. Some may be unaccustomed or resistant to staff assistance with eating and may push away either a hand or a spoon. They sometimes choke on either liquids or solid foods and need to be closely monitored while they eat.

Maintaining food consumption and adequate weight of residents with late-stage dementia may pose several challenges for staff. Most of these residents have severely impaired communication skills and cannot speak. Even in a one-to-one situation, they may have trouble comprehending cues, responding, and making their needs known. Short attention spans also make it hard for them to concentrate in a group dining setting. They are easily distracted from eating by whatever is going on around them in the dining room. Sensory deficits such as poor hearing and vision magnify these problems. The goal should be to simplify the setting so that they can better concentrate on the task at hand.

Interventions to Improve Eating

Communication

Before beginning to assist a resident to eat, staff should introduce themselves and let the resident know what will be taking place. For example, a nursing as-

Helping a Resident to Eat

Before offering a food item to a resident, explain what is being offered using adjectives such as *tasty, juicy,* and *delicious.*

Move your hand slowly toward a resident's mouth, offering a bite or a drink.

Let the resident know when a utensil is near his or her mouth.

Introduce the food gently by placing it on his or her lip.

Wait a minute to determine whether it is accepted or rejected by the resident.

If the resident rejects the food, then place a sweet-tasting item on the tip of a spoon; this may encourage the person to accept the food being offered. (Adapted from Otasz, 1986.)

sistant should approach a resident and say, "Hi, Mrs. Brown, I'm Sally and I'm going to help you eat your lunch. It's a cup of hot chicken soup and a cold turkey sandwich." Staff should sit down to assist residents rather than standing over them. Standing is authoritative and can make residents feel powerless. When assisting two residents simultaneously, a good strategy is to sit between them so that it will be possible to feed them in a leisurely, safe, and dignified manner.

Never force a person to eat. When a resident turns his or her head or says no, staff should not try to pressure the resident by forcing food or liquids into his or her mouth. This can be traumatic and cause the person to actively resist assistance or may produce a catastrophic reaction. If such struggles over eating occur repeatedly, they may worsen a resident's eating problem. As language abilities become further impaired, accurately understanding nonverbal cues from residents with dementia becomes important when assisting them in eating. Residents with difficulties expressing themselves verbally may have reasons that they cannot communicate to staff. For example, residents who have difficulties swallowing may instinctively turn their heads away when they are being fed too quickly. They may not have swallowed what is already in their mouths, and their refusing another mouthful of food is a way of protecting themselves from choking.

Staff need to learn alternative ways of communicating with residents, including interpreting body language, facial expressions, and other nonverbal cues. For example, residents may indicate that they want another bite by reaching for food or a utensil, opening their mouths, turning their heads, or raising their chins toward the person helping them. They may indicate that they do not want more food by spitting out food or refusing to accept a bite of food being offered. Staff also may cause rejection of food inadvertently by their own body language while assisting residents to eat. For example, moving away from the resident or talking to another staff member while offering food may cause rejection. Again, consistent staffing will help staff to become familiar with individual residents' eating patterns, remaining functional abilities, and preferences. Ostasz (1986) has provided additional hints for assisting a resident to eat.

Interventions for Problems with Chewing and Swallowing

A number of simple initial interventions may minimize residents' problems with chewing and swallowing. It may be enough to chop or cut food into small, bite-sized pieces and eliminate foods that are hard to chew, such as nuts, hard candy, popcorn, and raw carrots. Even foods such as cereal in milk can cause choking because the combination of a solid and liquid texture makes it difficult for residents with dementia to know whether to chew or swallow (Mace & Rabins, 1981). Also, foods that stick to the roof of the mouth (e.g., peanut butter) or have tough outer skins (certain types of fruit) should be avoided. These foods can easily become lodged in residents' throats, making them choke. Residents who do choke may become fearful of eating. As dementia progresses, it is better to serve these residents softer foods such as applesauce, cottage cheese, and scrambled eggs, which are easier to eat.

As choking problems become more severe, it may become necessary to grind, blend, or purée food before serving. Because soft foods provide more sensory stimulation for residents than puréed foods, they should be encouraged as long as they can be tolerated. Although a puréed diet may be easier for residents to eat, it is often uninteresting because it lacks an appealing shape, form, and texture; there is difficulty in visually identifying what type of food is being served; and the types of food that can be puréed lack variety. Residents who are switched to a puréed diet may lose weight as a result of both the monotony of the foods and the fact that it is usually implemented as dementia progresses. Food technology has improved, and products, such as Instant Pasta Puree, are available that more closely resemble the original foods (see "Where to Find Products" at the end of this chapter for sources).

Eventually, residents may cease to swallow even puréed foods and liquids. At this point, rapid weight loss may begin to occur. Using nutritional supplements to maintain adequate caloric intake can help increase total calories, protein, and fluid intake. Milkshakes, puddings, ice cream, and commercial supplements can be used effectively for this purpose. Extra snacks can be provided throughout the day, coupled with activity programming. Staff should monitor residents' fluid consumption closely and think of new ways to encourage increased consumption of fluids. Try to accommodate each person's preferences; if the resident does not enjoy water, offer juice or sweetened punch instead. Offer fluids throughout the day.

Handling Accidents

It is obvious that staff should not criticize residents' table manners, but it is also important to avoid subtly shaming residents (e.g., when food is spilled). Shaming can happen easily by staff's expressing annoyance over accidents at the table. For example, residents who spill food on the table or on their clothes may feel so upset or embarrassed by the incident and the staff reaction to it that they no longer feel like eating. When an accident does occur, staff should reassure the resident by quickly and calmly assisting with cleanup and providing new food or a clean plate for the person. Carefully consider seating arrangements and do not place residents who have difficulties eating next to others who will be critical of them and call attention to their problems.

Incorporating Food at Activities and Serving Special Meals

Food consumption need not be restricted to mealtimes. It may be easier to get some residents to eat snacks at activity programs than full meals at regular mealtimes. Activities often feature thematically appropriate foods to help orient residents to the activity (e.g., birthday cake). Residents may feel more in the mood to eat when they are attending a special event. After all, ice cream served at an ice cream social is much more exciting than ice cream served on a dinner tray.

Another way to make dining more pleasurable for residents is to make meals special events. These events can support residents' lifelong patterns. Even if residents are eating in the same dining room as usual, the room can be made to look and feel like something special is going to take place. For example, setting tables with white tablecloths and cloth napkins for a Sabbath meal is a familiar ritual for many older adults. Maintaining this routine may help orient some residents with dementia to the time of the week. Local clergy can come in and say a special prayer. Some residents may wish to invite family members to come and share this special meal with them.

Maintaining Residents' Dignity

Some residents may feel badly that they have difficulties eating neatly or may be worried about spilling food on their clothes. Yet they may find wearing a bib or a napkin at mealtimes child-like and demeaning. Finding adult solutions for these problems can help enormously. For instance, women may feel more comfortable wearing an apron or a smock to protect their clothes. Some residents also may prefer to wear an old cardigan sweater that can be easily laundered instead of a bib. Staff should be creative in finding solutions that are appropriate and maintain the dignity of these residents. (Adapted from Otasz, 1986.)

It is even more meaningful if the facility acquires favorite family recipes from its residents and prepares them for these special occasions. Ideally, residents can be involved in some or all aspects of the program by helping to prepare the food, decorate the dining room, and share their traditions.

When food is provided at an activity program, it should be served in a form in which residents can easily eat it. Prepare foods ahead of time so that residents will be successful in eating with less assistance. Do not serve food that is hard to handle (e.g., ice cream cones as opposed to the easier bowls of ice cream) and will upset residents if they drop it. Be especially sensitive to how food looks to residents with special dietary needs that prevent them from eating what others are having. For example, graham crackers served instead of a piece of birthday cake can be decorated to make them look as appealing as the cake. In addition, activity programs always should be used as an opportunity to offer more fluids, such as juice or lemonade.

Therapeutic Kitchens

Another way to encourage residents to eat is by holding cooking activities and, when possible, having a therapeutic kitchen. Many residents, especially women, have spent many hours preparing food in their home kitchens. Consequently, the kitchen is a familiar and comfortable environment for them. They may enjoy household activities, including washing dishes, setting tables, sweeping, and folding towels. Specific cooking activities that are popular include baking and decorating cookies, washing vegetables, and making bread. Therapeutic kitchens can provide a wonderful opportunity for residents to gather informally and socialize. Cooking together in the kitchen stimulates conversation by providing a common topic for those participating in the activity. Even residents with diminished verbal skills can have an enjoyable sensory experience while cooking. If possible, provide adequate kitchen workspace and ample seating room with several small tables and extra chairs.

Creating a therapeutic kitchen can be simple even if your facility does not have a place for cabinets, a sink, a stove, or a refrigerator. Some older adults may remember kitchens that centered around a large farmhouse-style table. The facility can purchase a table at which meals can be prepared and, if necessary, taken to the main kitchen to bake or cook. A baker's rack or an old cupboard can be added to the kitchen area. A countertop with cabinets can be accessorized with a canister set, potholders, a breadbox, and other kitchen-related items. If possible, add a refrigerator and sink later. A stove also may be added, but check with the local fire marshal before adding this appliance to determine if there are any restrictions.

WHAT THE ENVIRONMENT CAN DO

The physical setting is important to a pleasant dining experience. Good lighting, attractive decor, delicious smells, and quiet music create a relaxed mood for dining. Research studies show that eating in a calm, relaxing atmosphere in a long-term care facility can increase food consumption as well as mealtime socialization (Hall, 1994). Unfortunately, many aspects of the dining environment can cause problems for residents with dementia that may lead to excess disability. Changes to reduce or eliminate these problems are discussed later in this section. First, however, some suggestions are provided to help residents locate the dining room.

Finding the Dining Room

The first thing a resident must do before eating is find the dining room. This may seem simple, but it can prove to be a challenging task for some residents with dementia. Look at the facility through the residents' eyes:

- Do all of the room doors look the same?
- Is the same room used for all of the activities on the unit (including meals)?
- What makes mealtimes different or special as opposed to any other part of the day?
- Do meals arrive on covered trays, so that residents never get to smell the food before they are expected to start eating?

Residents with dementia are most likely to be able to identify the dining room and know it is time for a meal if this room is used only for meals or food-related activities. The facility may want to highlight the dining room door by painting it a bright color or using decorative moldings to call attention to it. If the dining room is a multipurpose room, then other sensory cues must be used to orient residents to mealtimes. These cues can be visual, such as setting the table with special colored linens and place mats or placing a large menu board in the hall. Cues also can be auditory, including playing the same piece of music each time prior to dining. Good smells such as bread baking or coffee brewing also are effective cues to draw residents to the dining room and stimulate their appetites. Tactile cues, including placing a napkin in a resident's hand, may help orient a person with dementia to mealtimes, as can sitting in the same seat in the dining room at each meal.

Minimizing Excess Disability

The dining rooms in many facilities create excess disability for residents with vision, hearing, and cognitive impairments. Many long-term care facility dining rooms are filled with glare and noise and hard surfaces, which are built-in distractions for residents with dementia. Administrators and designers often specify hard surfaces because they assume that those are easier to clean or will look cleaner. Cleanliness is an issue in the dining room; however, the facility also should consider residents' needs. Again, look at your dining room through the residents' eyes:

- Are large windows uncovered, letting in unfiltered bright sunlight?
- Are tabletops polished to a high gloss or topped with glass, reflecting bright light?
- Are the walls adorned with anything of interest?
- Would you want to eat every meal in this room?

These settings are unfamiliar and do not encourage residents to identify them with the experience of eating. By making a few changes that are supportive of residents, excess disability can be reduced and problematic behaviors decreased during mealtimes.

Room Size

An appropriately sized room for eating can make a big difference in the food consumption of some residents. The hurried, confusing, loud atmosphere in large institutional dining rooms can be overwhelming for residents with dementia. Small, crowded dining rooms where people are seated close together also can be distracting, and limit both independence and food consumption. Most residents are able to focus better on the task of eating when the dining room has a supportive atmosphere.

The best way to create a supportive atmosphere is to create several small dining rooms for 5–10 people. Smaller settings are more conducive to conversation and provide fewer distractions. Few facilities can afford this luxury; however, this effect can be achieved in multiple ways without building new dining rooms. Look for other spaces on the unit besides the dining room where residents who are easily distracted can eat. Because dining is a social occasion, however, residents should not eat alone unless that is their specific preference.

If only one room is used exclusively for dining, consider constructing permanent dividers (Figure 5.5). These can be short, attractively decorated

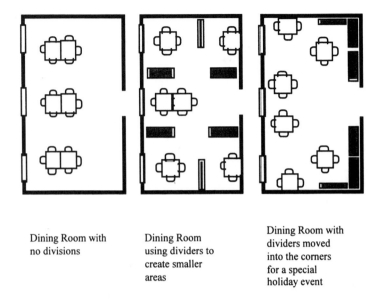

Dining Room with
no divisions

Dining Room
using dividers to
create smaller
areas

Dining Room with
dividers moved
into the corners
for a special
holiday event

Figure 5.5. Use permanent or moveable dividers to break a large
dining room into smaller sections to lessen distractions.

walls with planters or latticework depending on the style of the room. For design ideas, look at the ways in which large restaurants create small, intimate seating areas without dividing the space into small rooms. It is possible to divide the room into smaller areas temporarily if it is used for multiple activities. Moveable screens can be used to divide a large room into smaller areas. Screens can consist of standard shutters or panels found at most home decorating stores, or can be constructed using two-way hinges and shutters or pieces of plywood that can be decorated with cleanable padding and fabric or decoupage that residents can help create. Screens should be at least 5 feet tall to block vision and diffuse some sound.

If extra storage is needed, consider purchasing large cabinets with locking casters to divide the room (see "Where to Find Products" for sources). Standard wardrobe cabinets also can be used by affixing casters to them. The number of cabinets required is determined by the number of smaller "rooms" needed. These smaller areas should fit 5–10 people; you may want to consider having a smaller room for just two or three people. When the entire room is needed (e.g., for special holiday gatherings), the cabinets or screens can be pushed against a wall.

Decor

Decorating the eating areas with familiar objects and furnishings from residents' own homes can improve the level of social interaction. For older women especially, the kitchen and dining room were parts of their homes where they spent many hours. Therefore, these rooms often reflected their personal tastes and identities. The dining room is also a place where family heirlooms and treasures frequently are displayed. Many homes have a hutch or china cabinet filled with china, silver, or glassware that may have been handed down for generations. Consider placing a hutch in the dining room and filling it with china. Residents' families can be asked to donate some items, or china can be purchased at a garage sale or flea market. Some of the residents may enjoy tea parties served on this china from time to time.

Although it may not be possible to re-create a homelike dining room in a long-term care facility, attractive, homelike decor is likely to put residents in the mood to talk with one another and actually gives them an interesting subject about which to talk. When placing decorative objects, make sure that some are 4–5 feet above the floor where residents can see them.

Some psychology studies have attempted to determine what colors stimulate appetite in people. Although no studies have examined this issue specifically in people with dementia, some designers have suggested that "warmer, stronger colors in social dining rooms encourage conversation and interaction" (Brawley, 1997; p. 167). However, strong, bright colors may be too stimulating for some people. For this reason, Brawley encouraged the use of residential hues in the warm color range, including coral, peach, or soft yellows. Her book provides an extensive discussion of this subject and many other decorating issues for people in long-term care.

Designers and researchers do not always agree about the appropriateness of patterned materials such as wallcoverings, carpet, and fabric in rooms inhabited by people with dementia. Most designers believe that the absence of pattern in long-term care facilities contributes to their sterile image, whereas many researchers believe that bold, busy patterns can induce agitation in residents or create a confusing environment. To avoid either extreme, patterns must be selected carefully and placed in appropriate locations. The facility should avoid patterns that create visual distortions, such as large stripes or bold, repetitive patterns that contrast strongly with the background. Also, dominant patterns should be avoided in small rooms, particularly where they can be distorted by being reflected in a mirror. Patterns with highly contrasting colors on floor surfaces also should be avoided. Residents may interpret darker colors next to lighter colors as a step or a hole in the floor, causing a

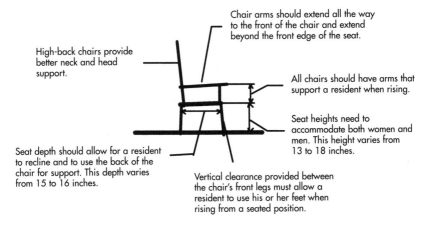

Chair arms should extend all the way to the front of the chair and extend beyond the front edge of the seat.

High-back chairs provide better neck and head support.

All chairs should have arms that support a resident when rising.

Seat heights need to accommodate both women and men. This height varies from 13 to 18 inches.

Seat depth should allow for a resident to recline and to use the back of the chair for support. This depth varies from 15 to 16 inches.

Vertical clearance provided between the chair's front legs must allow a resident to use his or her feet when rising from a seated position.

Figure 5.6.   Good dining room chair features.

loss of balance or confusion. If possible, avoid using a patterned surface as a backdrop for signs.

The best test for the appropriateness of patterns is the "squint test." When replacing any plain item of decor with a patterned version, insist on having a 3-foot-square sample. Squint at the pattern to see if any parts jump out at you or appear to move. Another strategy is to take a black-and-white photograph of the pattern or photocopy it on a black-and-white copier to see if there is any color that is brighter than the others, which could create distraction. With good planning, selection, and placement, a pattern can contribute to the interest created by an environment, but it must be chosen carefully.

Furniture

Dining Room Chairs

Chairs in dining rooms should support the seating posture that is the most conducive to eating and socializing (Figure 5.6). The distance from the chair to the table is also key for reducing excess disability. Residents become frustrated when they cannot easily see or reach the food on the table. All dining room chairs should have arms to provide a resting place for residents' arms, and make sure that the chair arms fit under the tables. This enables all residents, especially those with poor coordination or vision, to sit closer to the table so that they can better manage food and utensils.

The seat height and depth should allow residents to keep their feet on the floor and provide good lower back support. Younger people tend to sit forward while eating, whereas older people use the back of the chair for support to keep from slumping over. Excessive seat depths can make it difficult for older people to use the chair back for this purpose. Dining room chairs with tall backs provide additional support for the back and neck. Several chair manufacturers create seat heights that are a standard 18 inches above the floor. This height is too tall for many residents, and causes their feet to dangle above the floor. An older adult woman usually requires a seat height of 13–16 inches from the ground and a seat depth of between 16 and 18 inches. A typical older adult man requires a seat height of 18–19 inches and a seat depth of between 18 and 20 inches (Zavotka & Teaford, 1997). Keeping these numbers in mind, the facility should provide some chair variety for the residents to meet their different needs. One chair size rarely fits all residents. (See "Where to Find Products" for sources of a variety of dining room chairs.)

Experts have expressed different opinions on the benefits of having casters (wheels) on chairs. Placing casters on two of the chair legs make it easier for residents to pull up to and push away from the table. Having casters may reduce the staff effort that is required to assist residents with this activity. For high-functioning residents, casters may be a desirable feature; however, casters may make a chair unstable when a resident uses it for support. Therefore, they are not appropriate for unsteady residents. The facility should keep its residents' characteristics in mind when ordering chairs with casters. An alternative to casters is gliders, which are metal disks that glide easily over floor surfaces and can be attached to chair legs. Gliders are more stable than are casters.

Chairs also should have features that allow residents to sit as well as rise from a seated position easily. To enable residents to use chair arms for support when rising, the arms should extend to the front edge of the seat, and, if possible, extend slightly beyond the edge of the seat. Crossbars or panels between the front legs of a chair can make it difficult for residents to stand. To make it easier for an older person to stand, the area between the chair's front legs should have vertical clearance (e.g., no wood panel or crossbar). Stretchers, horizontal bars that run between the legs of chairs for stability, should be in the shape of an "H" rather than connect the bottoms of the legs forming a box. The area near the bottoms of the chair legs should be clear so that residents can effectively use their feet to push up from a seated position.

Dining Tables

When purchasing dining tables, the facility should keep the following issues in mind. Square tables are usually best because each resident is provided with his or her own side and "territory." A few two-person tables should be pro-

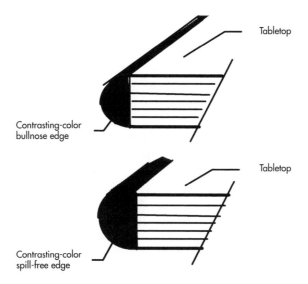

Figure 5.7.   Contrasting table edges.

vided for residents who benefit from fewer distractions. Bullnose edges on tables make resting residents' arms against them more comfortable and eliminate sharp edges that may cause an injury if someone falls. If the design calls for tables to be pushed together, then select edge treatments with few curves so that items (e.g., food, activity supplies) do not fall into the crevices. Similarly, make sure that the tables ordered do not have a decorative crevice between the edge and the table surface where crumbs can collect.

Using tables with contrasting edges make it easier for residents with low vision to distinguish the edges. Contrast can be achieved by using a different color or material (Figure 5.7). One additional benefit of purchasing a table with a contrasting edge is that the facility can specify the addition of spill-free edges to keep spilled liquids from dripping into residents' laps.

A wide array of table surface materials are available. Wood or wood laminates have a familiar, warm appearance, and it is easy to incorporate a contrasting edge on a laminate top. Whatever surface the facility chooses, a matte finish that does not reflect glare should be selected. In addition, the use of polishes or coatings on the tabletop, which are highly reflective, should be avoided.

Tables should be sturdy. Tables with four legs tend to be more stable than those with a center pedestal. However, center-pedestal tables are easier to use with wheelchairs because the table legs do not create an obstruction.

Some tables with four legs have an apron or a panel that extends along the underside of the tabletop between the legs. Make sure that chair arms fit under this apron. The bases of some center-pedestal tables can be adjusted for height to accommodate either wheelchair users and dining chair users. The typical table height is 29–30 inches from the floor, and most wheelchairs require 29 inches of clearance. This means that many wheelchairs will hit the edge of the table and users will not be able to pull up close enough to the table to eat. Therefore, a few adjustable-height tables are useful to include in a dining room (see "Where to Find Products" for sources).

Leveling tables so that they do not rock is often a problem because floors are rarely level. Many facilities resort to placing pieces of paper under the legs to keep tables stable. Tables that rock can be dangerous for residents who use tables for support. Both center-pedestal tables and tables with legs can be purchased with leveling features that alleviate this problem. The extra expense of leveling legs can be well worth it.

Flooring, Walls, and Ceilings

There are two broad categories of flooring that can be installed in dining rooms: carpeting and resilient flooring (Table 5.1). Carpeting can be area rugs or wall-to-wall carpets or carpet tiles, whereas resilient flooring can be sheet vinyl, vinyl composition tile, rubber flooring, or the like. Traditionally, most facilities have used resilient floors because they are easier to clean; however, resilient floors require more maintenance time than does carpeting. Carpeting has many benefits over resilient flooring, although resilient flooring can be cleaned more easily if spills occur frequently. Newer types of carpeting can withstand staining and maintain their appearance well. Because replacing a floor can be expensive, it is important to keep in mind all of these factors, not just the upfront costs. (See "Where to Find Products" for sources of carpeting and resilient flooring. See also Volume 4, Chapter 6 for further discussion of this topic.)

Walls are more than just a surface to be covered. Beyond contributing to the overall ambiance of the space, they affect residents' functioning in two significant ways: glare and reflected noise. Wall paint should have an eggshell finish, which is easier to clean than a matte finish. Gloss and semigloss finishes should be avoided because they reflect glare. Wallcoverings can transform an institutional-looking room to one that is much more residential in appearance. When selecting vinyl wallcoverings, the facility should choose a covering with either a matte finish or a delustered acrylic finish that will help to keep the surface clean. Several types of wallcoverings have sound-absorbing prop-

Table 5.1.   Comparison of carpeting and resilient flooring

	Carpeting	Resilient flooring
Preferred subfloor	Sealed concrete Odors can be trapped in unsealed floors, and liquids that penetrate may leach out if the subfloor is not sealed.	Sealed concrete Odors can be trapped into unsealed floors, and liquids that penetrate may leach out if the subfloor is not sealed.
Material forms	6–12 foot sheet carpet Carpet tiles	Sheet vinyl Vinyl composition tiles Sheet rubber
Maintenance procedure	Vacuum daily Periodically spot clean/extraction	Sweep and mop daily Periodically strip/Buff
Safety	Provides a cushion for falls Can still be walked on safely when wet Provides some resistance to feet of older people who shuffle when walking.	Can be slippery to walk on Some vinyl floors have added texture to increase traction. Very slippery to walk on when wet
Glare	Diffuses glare	Most resilient floors must be sealed with a polish to maintain their appearance. This polish is a source of glare. A few vinyl flooring products do not require such reflective coatings, and some coatings have less shine.
Noise reduction	Carpeting absorbs noise. Vacuums can have a decibel rating of 70–80 dB, which can disturb people on the unit, but some vacuums have a decibel rating of 50–60 dB. Extracting and spot cleaning cause a moderate amount of background noise.	Most vinyl floors reflect noise. Some rubber floors have sound-absorbing qualities. Sweeping and mopping are quiet ways of cleaning the environment.
Staining	With good-quality carpets, stains sit on top of the carpet fibers but should be spot cleaned as soon as possible.	Stains will be ground into the surface if not treated in a timely fashion.
Costs	More upfront costs to install; less expensive maintenance costs	Less expensive to install, but more costly to maintain

(continued)

Table 5.1. *continued*

	Carpeting	Resilient flooring
Appearance	Carpeting rarely wears out, but it can become worn if not maintained. Carpeting has a more residential appearance.	Resilient floors often have an institutional appearance. They are usually not found in dining rooms at home. A variety of resilient floor designs resemble the warm look of hardwood floors at a slightly higher cost.
Air quality	Independent studies have found that carpeting has the same air quality rating as hard surfaces with proper maintenance.	Resilient floors maintain good air quality if they are maintained properly.

erties (see "Where to Find Products"), but most have a porous finish and should be used sparingly where heavy staining is expected. Acoustical panels with a microperforated vinyl covering resists stains better. These wallcoverings can be used creatively as an accent wall instead of being placed on all of the walls in a room. Consider the use of drapes and other fabric window coverings, which provide some acoustical benefits at the windows as compared with shades or blinds.

Ceiling finishes also should be carefully selected in dining areas. Acoustical tile ceilings are common in most long-term care facilities. When replacement is necessary, try to find panels with the highest noise reduction criteria (NRC) possible. A good panel has a rating of 0.75 or higher; the higher the number, the better the rating. A drywall ceiling or soffit in the dining room can be given an acoustical spray finish that provides a textured look and reduces noise.

Lighting

Good lighting in the dining room is critical. Although changing the lighting can be expensive, it is often well worth the cost. The facility should examine whether the lighting in its dining room best suits its residents' needs and creates a pleasant atmosphere. (See Volume 1, Chapter 2 for more detailed information about types of lighting.)

Illumination levels must be distributed evenly about the room. In other words, all areas in the room should be of uniform brightness to reduce eyestrain caused by adapting to different conditions. To achieve this goal, indirect lighting is the best choice. Indirect lighting involves lighting fixtures that use the surrounding wall and ceiling surfaces to reflect light. Fixtures typically point up to distribute light across the entire ceiling surface. To supplement indirect lighting and to provide a warm residential appearance, the facility should incorporate chandeliers or wall sconces. A combination of direct and indirect lighting also improves residents' depth perception of objects. When lighting is too intense, shadows decrease and objects lose their impression of depth.

Dining rooms in long-term care facilities tend to be large, open rooms, often making them difficult to light well. To achieve good lighting, the proper fixtures should be used in the proper locations. If the dining room has standard fluorescent lights with acrylic lenses and the facility cannot afford to replace these fixtures, consider adding to them a parabolic reflector that will disperse the light in a less glaring pattern. Smaller grates that have openings that are 1-inch square or less are the most effective in controlling glare.

A facility that is considering replacing its fixtures should look at each room carefully first. Consider the ceiling height and the way in which the room will be used. If the ceiling height is just 8 feet, it is more difficult but still possible to use indirect lighting. Use a cove lighting scheme around the perimeter of the room for general illumination. Cove lights usually are built into ceilings or along walls and are often part of the architecture of the room. The facility can create a less expensive version of this lighting scheme by mounting a standard house gutter to the wall around the perimeter of the room at 6½–7 feet above the floor. Inside the gutter, mount strip fluorescent lights either on the wall or on the floor of the gutter (see Figure 5.8). After painting the gutter to match the wall or hanging a decorative border below the gutter, it will be impossible to tell that a gutter was used.

Chandeliers can be hung from an 8-foot-high ceiling if the furniture in the room will not be rearranged frequently. Chandeliers should properly be hung 30 inches above the table surface. Hence, if a room is to be used for multiple purposes, the facility should select a chandelier that hangs less than 1 foot below the ceiling. Rarely do chandeliers completely light a large room; therefore, these decorative fixtures always must be supplemented with other light sources.

Designers often prefer recessed can lights (downlights) because of their unobtrusive appearance on the ceiling, but these fixtures have limitations. Downlights disperse light evenly on a table surface when they are placed in a high ceiling (above 8 feet). If the ceiling height is less than 8 feet, down lights create pools of light on some tables while leaving other tables dark, unless they are spaced closely together. Downlights are best used as supplemental lighting and should not be the only form of lighting in a dining room. If

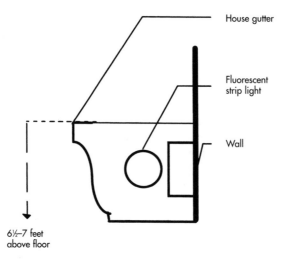

House gutter

Fluorescent
strip light

Wall

6½–7 feet
above floor

Figure 5.8.   House gutters and fluorescent lights can be
used to create an inexpensive version of cove lighting.

the dining room has a tall ceiling, use indirect light from chandeliers that
light the ceiling and provide some light directly on the tables below.

Wall sconces can supplement the lighting in a room or provide a decorative effect. If the facility chooses to use wall sconces to indirectly light a
room, a style that disperses light against the ceiling and the walls is best. Decorative wall sconces with chandelier-type bulbs can be used for decoration.
Make sure the wall sconces selected either do not extend more than 4 inches
from the wall or are hung 80 inches above the floor to satisfy the standards
set by the Americans with Disabilities Act of 1990 (ADA) (see "Where to Find
Products").

Color and Pattern

Older residents with low vision may have trouble distinguishing the food on
their plates, or the location of plates, glasses, and the like, if all are nearly the
same color. To improve this situation, serve foods of contrasting colors and
use simple table settings with strong color contrasts between table, place mats,
and plates. For example, a dark blue place mat under a white plate could be
used on a light-colored wood table. Highly visible borders around the edges
of the table and on the rims of cups and plates are also helpful. The facility
should choose patterns carefully (e.g., a heavily patterned tablecloth may af-

fect a resident's ability to concentrate on his or her plate). Color contrast between various foods on the plate also can stimulate residents' appetites. Try using differently colored garnishes, but remember that all garnishes that are served must be edible.

For residents who do not see well, staff should make sure that any assistive eating devices (e.g., silverware with high-contrast handles) are clearly in their view or are handed to them prior to eating. Residents will be more likely to use these devices if there is good color contrast between the handles of these implements and the color of the tabletop. When residents cannot see these devices, they are not likely to use them without staff cueing or assistance. It is also important to minimize clutter on the tables, both for residents who do not see well and for those who are distracted by clutter.

Utensils

Large-handled or modified utensils may help a resident to continue to eat more independently for a longer time. Putting out only the necessary silverware helps residents to make choices more easily. It is also helpful to serve a greater number of finger foods, which are easier for residents to eat. Other devices, such as rubber-coated spoons, can help older adults to avoid injuries that can occur when they bite down.

Using oversized dishes and cups may help residents to locate food and also help prevent spillage. Deeper rims sometimes can be enough to keep food from falling off plates. In some cases, bowls may be better than plates for residents who are embarrassed about spilling food, but this decision must be made on a case-by-case basis. As a last resort, plate guards also help prevent food from sliding off plates. A wet washcloth or a plastic place mat that grips the table surface may help keep the plate more stable on the table. A low-cost way to accomplish this is to buy a roll of safety strip material (e.g., similar to what is used under a throw rug to keep it in place) and cut out appropriate-size pieces to use under place mats (see "Where to Find Products").

Specially designed cups assist residents with poor grasp in holding these items. Covered or spouted drinking cups may permit low-functioning residents to drink independently, swallow better, and not spill liquids. Plastic travel mugs are both widely available and not childish in appearance. Their handles are often large and easy to hold, making them an excellent low-cost solution for some residents. Staff should customize interventions to be appropriate for each resident's current abilities. For example, do not give plastic car mugs to someone who can still use a ceramic coffee mug.

WHERE TO FIND PRODUCTS

Eating Aids

The following companies make a variety of assistive devices for eating, including plate guards, built-up utensils, and individual dishes:

AbilityOne Corporation
4 Sammons Court
Bolingbrook, IL 60440
(800) 323-5547
www.sammonspreston.com

AbleWare from Maddak, Inc.
661 Route 23 South
Wayne, NJ 07470
www.ableware.com, www.maddak.com

Alimed, Inc.
297 High Street
Dedham, MA 02026
(800) 225-2610
www.alimed.com

Extended Care Division (formerly Red Line HealthCare)
8121 10th Avenue North
Golden Valley, MN 55427
(800) 328-8111
www.redline.com

Skil-Care
29 Wells Avenue
Yonkers, NY 10701
(800) 431-2972
Slip-grip material in rolls that can be cut into the appropriate size for use under place mats

Cabinets for Dividing Dining Rooms

Adden Furniture, Inc.
26 Jackson Street
Lowell, MA 01852
(508) 457-7848

Allsteel, Inc.
Allsteel Drive
Aurora, IL 60507

(800) 764-2535
www.allsteeloffice.com
Allsteel's InterChange panel system consists of dividers with acoustical inserts on both sides. The company also offers a variety of wheeled cabinets for storage.

Furniture

Adjustable-Height Tables

Falcon Products, Inc.
9387 Dielman Industrial Drive
St. Louis, MO 63132-2214
(800) 873-3252
www.falconproducts.com
Access adjustable-height dining room table bases

Johnson Tables
1424 Davis Road
Elgin, IL 60123
(800) 346-5555

Kimball Lodging Group
1180 East 16th Street
Jasper, IN 47549-1009
(800) 451-8090
www.lodging.kimball.com
Health care and hospitality furniture

Space Tables
8035 Ranchers Road NE
Post Office Box 32082
Minneapolis, MN 55432-0082
(800) 328-2580
www.spacetables.com

Dining Room Chairs

HumanCare
14930 South Main Street
Gardena, CA 90248
(800) 767-4001
Human Care manufactures a variety of seating styles; custom seat heights can be special ordered

Lifespan
5901 Christie Avenue, Suite 101
Emeryville, CA 94608
(510) 601-6275
www.furnishings.com

Sauder Manufacturing
930 West Barre Road
Archbold, OH 43502-0230
(800) 537-1530
www.saudermanufacturing.com
Sauder offers a variety of health care-seating products.

Residential-Style Furniture

American of Martinsville
128 East Church Street
Martinsville, VA 24112
(540) 632-2061
www.americanofmartinsville.com

Basic American Medical Products
2935-A Northeast Parkway
Atlanta, GA 30360-2048
(770) 368-4700
www.basicamerican.com

Carroll Healthcare
1881 Huron Street
London, Ontario N5V 3A5
Canada
(800) 668-2337
www.carrollhealthcare.com

Duraframe
Post Office Box 1870
Ridgeland, SC 29936
(800) 405-3441
www.duraframe.com

Healthcare Furnishings, Inc.
31 Innwood Circle, Suite 109
Little Rock, AR 72211
(800) 648-5744
www.healthcarefurnishings.com

Invacare Continuing Care Group
739 Goddard Avenue
Chesterfield, MO 63005
(800) 347-5440
www.invacare-ccg.com

Kimball Healthcare
1600 Royal Street
Jasper, IN 47549-1001
(800) 482-1616
www.kimball.com

Primarily Seating
475 Park Avenue, Suite 3A
New York, NY 10022
(212) 838-2588
www.primarilyseating.com

Town Square
Post Office Box 419
Hillsboro, TX 76645
(800) 345-1663
www.gliderrocker.com

Flooring

Carpeting

Bonar Floors
365 Walt Sanders Memorial Drive
Newnan, GA 30265
(770) 252-4890
www.bonarfloor.com

Collins & Aikman Floorcoverings, Inc.
311 Smith Industrial Boulevard
Dalton, GA 30722-1447
(800) 248-2878
www.powerbond.com

Interface Flooring System, Inc.
Post Office Box 1503
LaGrange, GA 30241
(800) 336-0225
www.interfaceinc.com

Lees Commercial Carpets
3330 West Friendly Avenue
Post Office Box 26027
Greensboro, NC 27410
(800) 523-5647

Lowes Carpet Corporation
160 Duvall Road
Chatsworth, GA 30705
(800) 333-2468

Nonglare Resilient Flooring

Mannington Mills, Inc.
Post Office Box 30
Salem, NJ 08079
(800) 356-6787
www.mannington.com
Their Custom Spec II sheet vinyl line has a heavier sealer coat that does not require shiny polish. Colors and patterns have low contrast, and two patterns imitate a hardwood floor. Costs are only slightly higher than those of standard vinyl.

TOLI International
55 Mall Drive
Commack, NY 11725
(800) 446-5476
www.toli.com
Vinyl sheets and vinyl tile that are extremely durable and a variety look like hardwood floors. These products also have less sheen compared with other vinyl. Their Spectrafloors line is a textured product that, when left unpolished, diffuses glare. Costs are higher than for standard vinyl flooring, but the product is considered more durable.

Quiet Vacuum Cleaners

Windsor Industries, Inc.
2351 W. Standford Avenue
Englewood, CO 80110
(303) 762-1800, (800) 444-7654
Manufactures Windsor Sensor, an upright vacuum cleaner for institutional use. This vacuum is rated at 69 dB at the operator, which is the

sound level of normal conversation. At 10 feet away, the sound level of the vacuum drops to 62 dB.

North American Cleaning Equipment
Distributed by Newport Equipment Co., Inc.
24857 Broadway Avenue
Bedford, OH 44146
(440) 439-2224
Manufactures NVQ 402, a tank vacuum for institutional use. This vacuum is rated at 50 dB at the operator, which is well below the sound level of normal conversation.

Acoustical Wall Treatments

Conwed Designscape
800 Gustafson Road
Ladysmith, WI 54848
(800) 932-2383
www.conweddesignscape.com

Illbruck Architectural Products
3800 Washington Avenue North
Minneapolis, MN 55412
(800) 225-1920
www.illbruck-archprod.com

JM Lynne Co., Inc.
59 Gilpin Avenue
Post Office Box 1010
Smithtown, NY 11787
(800) 645-5044
www.jmlynne.com
Flame-retardant acoustical textile wallcoverings

Pyrok Inc.
121 Sunset Road
Mamaroneck, NY 10543
(914) 777-7070
www.pyrokinc.com

Other acoustical companies can be found at *www.constructionmaterials. com*. This web site has an extensive list of companies that manufacture acoustic wall treatments.

Lighting

ADA–Compliant Wall Sconces

SPI Lighting, Inc.
10400 North Enterprise Drive
Mequon, WI 53092
(414) 242-1420
www.spilighting.com
Their Phaces wall sconces meet ADA's 4-inch clearance standard and come with a variety of lighting options.

Lighting Consultants

Eunice Noell-Waggoner
Center for Design for an Aging Society
6200 S.W. Virginia Avenue, Suite 210
Portland, OR 97201
(503) 246-8231
Noell-Waggoner is an expert in the field of lighting for aging people.

Illuminating Engineering Society of North America
120 Wall Street, Floor 17
New York, NY 10005
(212) 248-5000
www.iesna.org
Lighting and the Visual Environment for Senior Living (1998).

Lighthouse International
111 East 59th Street
New York, NY 10022-1202
(800) 829-0500
www.lighthouse.org
Lighthouse International offers a variety of solutions and products for individuals with visual impairment.

◆◆◆

A summary sheet follows, which condenses the chapter text into a quick overview. The authors have also provided an area for you to make your own notes about your own staff and facility. Managerial staff may wish to use the summary sheets as handouts to accompany direct care staff training, or to post them by the time clock or nurses' station or include them in staff's pay envelopes.

EATING SUMMARY SHEET

1. Eating food is more than simple nutritional intake; it is a symbol of nurturing. Eating is usually integral to the rituals of holidays, life celebrations, and special events.

2. Eating is highly individualized in the number of meals eaten per day, places in which each person likes to eat, size of meal, time of day, seating, service style, type of food and food preferences, temperature, table setting, background music, and so forth.

3. Residents of long-term care facilities may eat poorly because of changes in portion size/food type, reduced ability to smell or taste, poor vision/hearing, embarrassment, anxiety, depression, mouth pain, hand dexterity problems, gastrointestinal problems, or association of particular foods with unhappy events.

4. Residents with dementia may not correctly identify feelings of hunger or recognize food or utensils, may have difficulty finding the dining area, may have difficulty concentrating when the environment is noisy or if table companions converse intensely, or may have chewing/swallowing difficulties.

What Staff Can Do

1. Help residents maintain dignity by avoiding embarrassing or childish approaches—avoid using bibs or cutting their food in front of them at the table. Handle spills quietly and matter-of-factly. Make sure that table companions are appropriate according to both functional and social levels as well as compatible personalities.

2. Maintain familiar routines and support individual preferences. Provide familiar cues. Observe individual texture/temperature/condiment likes and dislikes.

3. Serve foods in typical courses/ways and identify them for residents each time.

4. Create and maintain a pleasant atmosphere for dining, provide at least some finger foods, serve food "on the run," use the 5 Ws to analyze eating problems.

5. Maintain settings/traditions/rituals that reflect weekend and holiday meals.

6. Encourage resident participation in food/table preparation or baking activities.

What the Environment Can Do

1. Clearly mark paths/entry to the dining room, and use aromas to attract people.

2. Eliminate glare, avoid crowding and confusion, and create small dining clusters.

3. Make the dining room a familiar and attractive place to eat. Select soft and warm colors, comfortable patterns, chairs/tables that support ease in eating, attractive flooring and wallcoverings, and adequate/appropriate lighting. Use sound-deadening materials wherever possible.

4. Select dishes with contrasting borders that also contrast with table surfaces and table cloths. Avoid the use of strong patterns. Use edible garnishes to make plates attractive

5. Provide appropriate adaptive dishes and utensils.

YOUR NOTES

6

Dressing

In American culture, looking good is linked to a person's sense of well-being and self-esteem. Like it or not, we often make judgments about people based on their appearance. Consequently, many people spend considerable time thinking about what they wear. Most people, however, never think about what it would be like if they regularly experienced difficulty getting dressed. For most of us, dressing is a simple and quick procedure that we go through one or even several times per day. Rarely do we stop to consider all of the different steps involved in getting dressed.

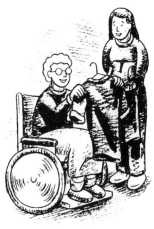

Dressing can be a serious problem and cause frustration for people who have physical or cognitive deficits or both that affect their ability to do this task. This section discusses the personal impact of not being able to dress independently, reasons why older adults are likely to experience these difficulties, and ways to minimize these problems.

WHEN OLDER ADULTS HAVE TROUBLE DRESSING

Older adults' sense of self-identity is affected when they have trouble maintaining their appearance as they would like. For instance, if Mr. Miller has arthritic hands, he may not be able to tie the knot in his necktie properly or button his shirt. If Mrs. Roth has a tremor in her hands, she may have trouble fastening her bra or applying her makeup evenly. Sometimes older people compensate by simply changing the way in which these tasks are accomplished. For instance, Mr. Miller might start wearing a clip-on bow tie, or Mrs. Roth might buy a makeup brush that is easier to grip. Older people may devise these solutions themselves or they may seek advice from others about new ways to accomplish these familiar tasks.

Sometimes the dressing problems of older adults are more serious, and these individuals require greater physical assistance with dressing. Having difficulties in completing ADLs such as dressing is a common reason why older people move into a more supportive environment, such as assisted living. Despite needing this help, some residents may feel that having staff assist them with dressing is embarrassing and an invasion of their privacy. Many older people are easily embarrassed by being naked in front of others; this generation grew up in an era when modesty was highly prized. It is not surprising, therefore, that many older people find receiving this type of personal assistance to be unfamiliar, hard to accept, and, in some cases, frightening. However, changes in both physical and cognitive functioning often make such assistance necessary.

PHYSICAL ISSUES

As people age, they may develop certain physical problems that affect their ability to get dressed easily. These may include mobility problems, sensory impairments, and increased frailty. The following discussion briefly summarizes both physical and cognitive issues that have an impact on individuals' ability to dress.

Certain diseases to which older people are more prone, including arthritis, stroke, and Parkinson's disease, can cause significant mobility problems that affect the ability to dress. Decreased muscle strength or control, restricted range of motion, coordination problems, impaired gait, and poor balance all can affect dressing ability. (For a more extensive discussion of mobility problems, see Chapter 3 in this volume.) Many older people become easily tired, and those who have multiple health problems may have even more trouble performing their activities of daily living (ADLs). Therefore, they may be able to do only a certain number of tasks effectively during the day. Just getting dressed may require them to use a significant amount of their physical and mental energies. Simplifying the dressing process may give them more stamina to do other things, such as eating meals and participating in activities.

Age-related sensory impairments also can make it harder for an older person to dress independently. Too often, problems related to sensory losses are simply attributed to the resident's being confused or showing signs of dementia. Impaired vision can have a significant effect on a resident's ability to select appropriate clothes, locate these garments in a closet or chest of drawers, and figure out how to put them on correctly. Residents with low vision easily may make mistakes such as wearing a shirt inside out or selecting two different-colored socks. A diminished sense of touch can make it much harder for these residents to put on clothing successfully and correctly fasten buttons or close snaps.

DIFFICULTIES OF DRESSING FOR RESIDENTS WITH DEMENTIA

For residents with dementia, both mental and physical impairments can make it even harder to dress independently. Because of their combined perceptual, cognitive, and motor problems, these residents often have problems with various stages of dressing. People with dementia vary in the levels of both cognitive impairment and physical disabilities that affect their ability to dress independently. Not all residents with dementia are impaired equally at the same stages of dementia. Some residents remain able to dress independently, some require only verbal or physical cueing or both, and others may need complete assistance (Beck, 1988).

A number of different cognitive problems may affect in specific ways an individual's ability to dress. Certain residents may have trouble sequencing steps in dressing, whereas the cognitive problems of other residents may be related to starting the physical motions of getting dressed (Beck, 1988). Specific ways to assist residents with each of these types of problems are discussed in "What Staff Can Do." Cognitive deficits coupled with sensory losses may significantly worsen dressing problems. To illustrate, the combination of limited sight and confusion makes it more difficult for residents to select and put on appropriate sequences of clothing. Poor hearing also can make it more difficult to communicate with and give verbal instructions to residents who need step-by-step cueing in getting dressed.

WHAT STAFF CAN DO

Understanding Residents' Feelings

Staff should always keep in mind that, even for residents with dementia, it is often frustrating or embarrassing to need help dressing. Be sensitive to how residents may feel when you are helping them to get dressed. Try to imagine yourself in the resident's position. To gain a better understanding of this, staff should practice helping each other put on clothes and do other kinds of personal care, such as washing each other's feet. It is likely that most will find this sensitivity exercise highly embarrassing and uncomfortable, but this is one of the best ways to learn about how residents may feel when they receive this type of personal care.

Because dressing is such a highly personal experience, it is important to provide residents with as much privacy as possible. When residents need step-by-step cueing, staff may be able only to step back a bit or turn their backs while the residents are doing the most personal aspects, such as putting on underwear. When residents just need to have their clothes selected, staff may be able to provide them with more privacy. For example, staff can lay out the clothes and then leave to assist others, returning to check whether the resident needs any additional assistance. Most people are more comfortable with members of the same gender when it comes to personal care such as help getting dressed.

Residents who have had disfiguring or scarring surgeries (e.g., mastectomies, colostomies, burns) may be self-conscious about their scars or other changes to their bodies. It is particularly important to provide adequate privacy for these residents. One way to do this is to drape the affected parts of their bodies with a towel or sheet while they are dressing to help maintain their dignity. Even residents with dementia may care deeply and be highly sensitive about these issues. Think about how you would feel in their position and how you would want to be treated.

Taking a Therapeutic Approach

Each resident's ability to dress should be assessed so that strategies can be devised to maximize their remaining functional abilities. Even if it is more time consuming for residents to dress independently, there are significant therapeutic benefits in doing so. Staff should try not to cause excess disability by always doing things for residents but instead let them accomplish tasks themselves. This is especially important for residents with dementia because skills can be lost rapidly if others do everything for them. Staff can make the process of dressing easier for these residents in a number of ways. Although initially it may seem time consuming to implement these strategies, this therapeutic approach may result in savings in staff time required for assistance.

How to Evaluate Dressing Ability

As with the assessment of many other ADLs, assessment of dressing is often broken down into the following three categories: 1) total independence, 2) partial independence, and 3) total dependence. Table 6.1 shows some of the characteristics of residents commonly classified in each of these categories. Although these classifications are a useful starting point, staff should not use these labels exclusively to determine a resident's capabilities. It is important to maintain a flexible, open-minded attitude about what individual residents can accomplish. Dressing is a complex task, and there are a wide variety of cognitive impairments that may result in an individual's having difficulty completing the task. For example, an individual with *ideational apraxia* may have problems organizing the sequence of dressing, whereas an individual with *ideomotor apraxia* may not be able to make the necessary movements required for dressing (Beck, 1988). One of the important points noted in Beck's article is that excess disability is often created for individuals with dementia when caregivers do things for people instead of letting them do the task for themselves. By determining the particular aspect of the task with which the individual is having difficulty, it is often possible to make adaptations to the task so that the person can continue to complete some of the task on his or her own. Beck (1988) developed a useful ADL assessment scale (the Beck Dressing Performance Scale) that specifically evaluates both the physical and cognitive aspects of dressing and looks at the level of assistance that is needed from the caregiver.

Using the 5 Ws to Evaluate Dressing Abilities

The multipurpose 5 Ws—who, what (e.g., what behavior), where, when, and why—introduced earlier in this volume also can be helpful in solving dressing problems. In addition to the Beck Dressing Performance Scale, the 5 Ws provide a way of thinking about how different factors, including staff and environmental features, may enhance or hinder residents' ability to dress more

Table 6.1.   Levels of dependence in dressing

Total independence	Partial independence	Total dependence
Can select appropriate clothes	Can select clothes with some assistance	Needs complete assistance in dressing
Can put on own clothes, including socks and shoes	Can put on clothes with either physical or verbal assistance from staff	
Can perform dressing tasks requiring fine motor skills (e.g., closing buttons, zippers)	May be able to perform some tasks requiring fine motor skills, such as closing snaps or Velcro fasteners	

Adapted from Eliopoulos (2000).

independently. (The 5 Ws are discussed as a part of the Behavior Tracking Process in Volume 3, Chapter 1. The Behavior Tracking Form can be found in Appendix A of that volume as well.)

The first phase of the assessment of dressing is thinking about why a particular resident is having trouble getting dressed. Staff should watch him or her perform the entire task and make notes regarding what types of assistance he or she needs. The Beck Dressing Performance Scale can be used to evaluate the specific stages at which the resident is having difficulties. Then staff should think about who is generally assisting the resident and what types of help are being provided. Next, staff should consider what else is going on in the environment that may be hindering the resident's ability to focus on the task at hand (e.g., loud music playing on the radio may be affecting his or her ability to concentrate). Also, they should determine where the problems are occurring: Is the resident having trouble selecting clothes from the closet, or having problems physically putting them on because he or she is losing his or her balance while trying to dress? Finally, staff should consider when the resident experiences the most difficulties with dressing. Like other people, a resident with dementia has good and bad days. He or she sometimes may be able to dress more independently and at other times may require more assistance. If the resident has not slept well and is tired or in pain, it may be hard for him or her to concentrate on getting dressed. At these times, the person may require more time or additional assistance in getting ready.

Staff who regularly help residents with dressing problems should implement a tracking process to evaluate when problems occur. They can keep the tracking forms in a handy location such as taped inside a closet door. This is both private and easily accessible for staff to make notes. Certain residents may become upset that staff are jotting things down while watching them dress. In such cases, staff should make mental notes and write the information on the tracking forms later. It is more important to be sensitive to the residents' feelings and not upset them while they are performing this task than it is to write down information about them.

After you have gathered information by observing residents dress, talking to family and other staff, reading the residents' charts, and possibly getting a professional assessment from an occupational or a physical therapist, staff can proceed to the next step. Analyze the information that has been collected to determine whether there are simple steps that can be taken to make the dressing process easier for these residents. Because each resident's cognitive and physical abilities may change over time, staff must continually monitor and evaluate how well each strategy is working. If a strategy does not work any longer, then staff must try to think of new solutions to address the problem.

Stages of Dressing

There are several stages of dressing for which staff should consider ways to help residents with dementia to dress more independently. These include helping residents with

- Selecting clothing
- Sequencing clothing
- Performing the physical steps of dressing

The following text considers in detail how staff can help residents with each of these important issues.

Selecting Clothes

Too often, living in a long-term care facility greatly restricts people's ability to make their own choices. Selecting what to wear is an important way in which people can express themselves (Figure 6.1). Being able to perform this simple task can help residents to maintain their self-identity and self-esteem. After all, it is psychologically beneficial for residents to look and feel their best.

Asking residents what they like to wear and looking at pictures of how they dressed when they lived at home can provide opportunities for good conversations with residents to reminisce about fashionable clothes. You may make Mrs. Bloom's day by listening to her story about the dress that she wore on her first date with her husband. Similarly, you may learn that wearing a baseball cap reminds Mr. Haverty of his days in the minor leagues and is a source of happiness for him. When residents have trouble communicating verbally, ask family members about how they dressed and record this information in the social history section of their charts.

Social norms about dressing were different when residents were young. This generation dressed more formally, especially when they went out in public. For instance, women commonly wore hats and gloves when they went to church. Men wore suits and ties to the office on a daily basis, not just for meetings. Because our dressing style today is much more casual than in the past, it may be difficult for residents with dementia to recognize themselves when wearing a jogging suit or a pullover and jeans. They may be confused not only because of dementia but also because they do not identify with the images they now see in the mirror.

To the greatest extent possible, staff should help each resident to preserve his or her personal dressing habits. Some residents have always been more concerned about how they look than others have. Try to learn how each

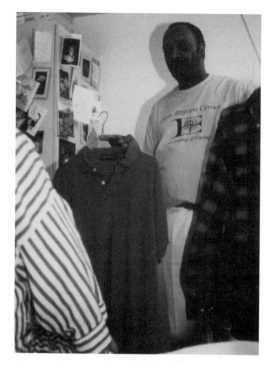

Figure 6.1. Helping residents with dementia to select their clothing can contribute to their self-esteem.

resident feels about these issues and take their personal needs into consideration. Even if it is more practical for residents to dress casually, some men may not feel like themselves without a tie and some women may not feel properly dressed without wearing makeup and having their hair done.

Little things can make a big difference in terms of how a resident with dementia feels about him- or herself. A woman who always wore a lot of jewelry will appreciate having a nice pin or two to wear on her outfit every day. Using the same perfume that she has always worn also may help her to feel connected with her life before the onset of dementia. Scheduling a weekly visit to the beauty parlor for some older women may help to reinforce their previous routines, sense of time, and continuity of self. It does not take much extra staff time to implement these small personal touches that can mean so much to the residents.

Sometimes residents with dementia may select unusual or inappropriate combinations of clothing. It is important to understand that there may be reasons why residents choose what they are wearing. Some may be physical; the resident may be cold and want the extra layers for warmth. Some inappropriate choices may be due to sensory problems; for example, a resident may have difficulty seeing the clothes he or she has selected. An agenda behavior approach may help staff to understand the choices that residents may be making. *Agenda behavior* is the planning and behavior that residents use in an attempt to meet their social, emotional, or physical needs at a given time (Rader, Doan, & Schwab, 1985). This approach, which was developed by three nurse researchers, suggests that people typically do things for a reason. Thus, it is important to attempt to determine why the resident is doing something before you try to change that behavior. (A detailed description of the agenda behavior approach can be found in Volume 3, Chapter 1.) For example, if Mrs. Lee's vision is impaired, she may be picking out clothes that she thinks are a matching set when they are not. Staff should be sensitive in determining whether she made a mistake or her choice was intentional. After all, it may be her personal taste to wear these two items together, in which case her wishes should be honored regardless of how others think that the outfit looks.

Sometimes a person with dementia may want to wear the same outfit every day. This may be because he or she does not remember wearing it on the previous day. There may be something about the color or style that makes it easier for the resident to see, or perhaps he or she really likes the outfit and is attracted to it in the closet. If it is hung in the same position in the closet, that spot may be the one that the resident sees best, and therefore he or she always chooses it. Also, in some cultures, people are used to wearing the same clothes for several days in a row. They may not have had the opportunity to wash clothes as frequently as we do today, or they may have been poor and only owned a limited amount of clothing. Remember that this cohort of older people was influenced by the Great Depression, and they are used to saving and making things last as long as possible. Therefore, they may choose to keep wearing the same clothes and save those that are newer in their closet for special occasions. Sometimes they may never get around to wearing the new clothing.

When residents choose to wear the same clothes, it is important to be patient and treat them with respect and dignity. Staff should avoid confrontations over this issue so that the residents do not become combative during dressing and develop negative feelings about this daily ritual. Try to wash the favorite clothes often so that they are clean and available for the resident to wear. If possible, these clothes should be removed from the closet for cleaning when the resident is not present (e.g., if the resident goes to the dining room for a meal). Another option is to ask the family to supply multiple sets of favorite outfits or garments that are the resident's favorite color. If a resident consistently wanders into another resident's room and takes specific garments, then staff should try to determine the agenda behind this behavior so that appropriate interventions can be developed.

> *Mrs. Kasabian continually went into Mrs. Anderson's room and removed a sweater decorated with sequins and put it on. This made Mrs. Anderson angry because the sweater was a birthday present from her granddaughter. She usually lost her patience and yelled at Mrs. Kasabian, calling her a thief. On several occasions, she even tried to pull the sweater off Mrs. Kasabian's back. When staff realized that the problem was related to this specific garment, they spoke to Mrs. Kasabian's family and recommended that they buy her two similar sequined sweaters to wear. After Mrs. Kasabian received her own sweaters and staff offered her one to wear every morning, she stopped taking Mrs. Anderson's sweater. Making available two similar sweaters for Mrs. Kasabian prevented the problem from occurring even on days when one of the sequined sweaters was being laundered.*

Sequence of Dressing

Many residents with dementia experience problems with the sequence of putting on clothes that are directly related to their cognitive deficits. In some cases simplifying the process of dressing can help reduce these problems. Tasks for people with short-term memory problems must be broken down into steps that can be done one at a time. A series of discrete steps help residents to focus on a single aspect of dressing at a time.

When a resident opens the closet door, choosing among his or her garments may be overwhelming because too much visual information is being presented at once. This can affect memory and make it hard for him or her to know how to proceed. Offering a limited number of choices can help a resident to make a selection while still having control over deciding what he or she wants to wear. Organizing clothing by color or type can help residents with dementia, low vision, or both to make appropriate selections more easily. Some facilities have done research using specially designed closets. For example, at the Corrine Dolan Alzheimer Center, one study showed that independence in dressing could be increased by 19% using a specially modified closet (Namazi & Johnson, 1992a). In this closet, only one set of clothes was visible, hung in the correct order for dressing. This helped the resident to put on the clothes sequentially (e.g., underwear before pants). This arrangement reduced the need for direct physical assistance by one third to one half. More people were able to dress with only verbal prompts using this closet system. This scheme helped them to focus on one aspect of dressing at a time and ultimately made them less reliant on caregivers for physical assistance with dressing. (See "What the Environment Can Do" for information on re-creating this closet.)

If you cannot make a specially designed closet, then the same effect can be achieved by installing a multiple-hanger rack that goes over the door and holds the clothes in the right order for dressing. Some residents may need to have only one set of clothes removed from the closet and laid out in order on the bed. Similarly, placing the residents' socks on top of their shoes helps them to put these items on in order. Keep trying different arrangements until you find one that works best for each resident. For example, a shorter resident may do better when the clothes are hung over the back of a chair rather than on the closet door so that they are easier to reach.

Furthermore, not all people get dressed in the same order. Staff should interview close family members (e.g., a resident's spouse) to find out each resident's patterns while getting dressed. For example, if Mr. Norman always put on his socks following his underwear or right before his shoes, then keeping his routine consistent will help him to be able to put on his clothes sequentially. Would you find it easy to change a pattern that you have been following every day for 75 years?

At home, Mrs. Harper always kept her underwear in the top right dresser drawer and her stockings in the top left drawer. However, these items were arranged in the wrong order in her dresser at the facility. Staff noticed that she often had trouble finding her stockings in the morning. After talking with her daughter, they switched the arrangement of the items and labeled her dresser drawers with large, easy-to-read labels. After making these simple changes, Mrs. Harper was able to dress more independently. She expressed to her daughter that she felt good about no longer having to ask staff to help her find her stockings every morning.

Another technique that may be effective with some residents is to make dressing cards with a simple picture and text showing a person performing the next step required. This picture may help residents to remember what they are supposed to do next by reinforcing the verbal cue. This can be particularly helpful for residents who have impairments in receptive language (understanding verbal directions), problem-solving, or sequencing skills. Make sure that the dressing cards are large enough so that residents can see the pictures and text easily and that the cards have good color contrast. Each card should demonstrate one step of the activity using both a picture and simple words to describe the step it represents. The instructions should be written or typed in large letters that are easy to read. Written cues to accompany the pictures are important because many individuals with dementia maintain the ability to read words well into the late stage of dementia (Bayles & Tomoeda, 1995; Brush & Camp, 1998).

In a set of sequencing cards for dressing, the first card might show a resident in nightclothes. The second card could show the day's clothes being laid out on the bed in the order in which they will be put on, the third could show staff assisting with taking off the nightclothes, the fourth could show staff assisting with putting on the day's clothes, and the last card could show the resident dressed and smiling. Staff can either lay the cards on a nearby surface (e.g., bed, dresser, bathroom counter) or hand the cards to the resident one at a time. Staff then point to each card in the sequence and have the resident read the step to determine whether he or she understands what it means.

Sequencing cards can be made or purchased. Speech therapists use sequencing cards with clients to facilitate communication. You may want to seek a referral to a speech-language pathologist for residents with impaired communication abilities. Occupational therapists also use sequencing cards to facilitate communication during ADLs. If it is not possible to work with one of these professionals, there are a variety of ways to create sequencing cards (see "Where to Find Products" at the end of this chapter for sources). Therapy supply catalogs carry products that can be used to make the cards. "Pick 'n Stick" are packages of color stickers that depict a variety of subjects. Board-Builder and Boardmaker are computer programs that help staff to design communication displays. These programs offer 3,000 symbols to choose to create custom cards. Premade sequencing cards manufactured by Winslow Press can be purchased through therapy supply catalogs, but these cards do not have word instructions included. Finally, staff can create cards using photographs or pictures cut out of catalogs or sales books. Laminate the cards so that they will not be damaged by water.

Physical Act of Dressing

The physical steps involved in getting dressed also may cause problems for residents with both cognitive and physical impairments. Some types of clothing are easier for certain residents to put on depending on the nature of their physical disabilities (e.g., pullover versus button-down shirts). For residents with dementia, there is also the issue of what kinds of clothes they are most familiar with wearing. For example, some older women may have always worn blouses that buttoned down the front. However, blouses on which the buttons are hidden under a flap of material may be extremely confusing to them. Some residents can continue wearing the same styles of clothing but switch to versions that are easier to put on independently (e.g., elastic-waist pants and skirts). Velcro fasteners are easier to manipulate than zippers, buttons, and snaps, but they are less familiar to older people. Some other devices that are easier to manipulate include large-ring or loop-handled zippers or button-hooks. (See "Where to Find Products" for a list of sources for dressing aids.)

Shoes also should be easy to put on and remove. Most residents with dementia do better with slip-on styles. Those who can still walk should wear shoes that provide adequate support. Tennis shoes or other shoes with crepe soles also may help to prevent falls.

Some residents with mobility problems may require greater physical assistance in getting dressed. A professional evaluation from an occupational or physical therapist may be needed to determine what types of adaptive equipment are most beneficial for residents who have problems bending and reaching. Such an evaluation is likely to include assessment of the resident's muscle strength and tone, range of motion, and cognitive status. It is also important to find out what else is going on in the environment that may be distracting or may make it difficult for a resident with both dementia and mobility problems to get dressed. For example, if a radio is playing, then it may be harder for the resident to focus on dressing, and he or she may experience additional difficulties in maintaining balance and coordination.

It is worth thinking about how to adapt regular clothes for residents who spend most or all of their time in a wheelchair, both to ensure their privacy and to provide greater comfort. It is especially important to supply clothing that is loose fitting, particularly around the waist and hips, so that it is comfortable and less binding. Families can help by selecting clothing for their loved ones that is loose fitting and comfortable and suits their style. Andresen (1995) recommended that fabrics be lightweight and flexible and feel soft against the resident's skin. This is especially important for residents with impaired mobility and those who sit in chairs for most or all of the day. Clothing also should be durable, washable, flame retardant, and easy to put on.

How It Feels to Need Help Getting Dressed

As residents with dementia become more cognitively impaired, they often require greater assistance in getting dressed successfully, but they may not perceive the need for help and be resistant when staff attempt to provide assis-

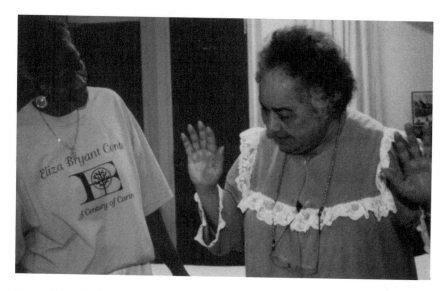

Figure 6.2.   Residents can become upset when they need assistance with dressing.

tance. From a young age, most people are not used to receiving any assistance with dressing. Therefore, it can be unfamiliar and disturbing for residents with dementia to need help in completing this familiar task. Staff should not to take it personally when residents become angry while they are assisting them; they probably are more frustrated with the situation than with staff (Figure 6.2).

Mr. Gudnicki is an independent man with early-stage Alzheimer's disease. He does not respond well when he receives dressing assistance from female nursing assistants. He becomes quite upset, yells, and sometimes throws his clothes. By observing him, staff found that he is able to dress more independently when he has more time in the morning to get ready. From his social history, staff know that he was a factory worker who left for the plant at 5:00 A.M. every day. They interviewed his wife and learned that he was an early riser; even on weekends he never got up later than 5:30 A.M. Knowing this, the night staff decided to wake him at 5:00 A.M. to give him extra time to get dressed in the mornings. They started a new routine of helping him to select his clothes and lay them out the night before so that he would not have this extra pres-

*sure in the morning. Because Mr. Gudnicki was used to dress-
ing casually, staff recommended that his family buy him new
clothes that were easier to put on (e.g., comfortable sweats,
tennis shoes with Velcro closures). This enabled him to dress
more independently, which made him much happier. Also,
it was indicated in his chart that he should always be paired
with a male staff member to assist him in getting dressed.
Once these changes were made, Mr. Gudnicki was able to
dress more independently and stopped being combative in the
mornings.*

Some residents may have a catastrophic reaction during personal care.
When this happens first thing in the morning, they may be too upset to eat
breakfast or enjoy a morning activity that they normally like. Routinely having problems with dressing can be both tiring and stressful for residents.
Stress can have negative consequences on physical health, including elevated
heart rate and blood pressure and increased agitation in residents. Therefore, staff should brainstorm ways to minimize the dressing problems of individual residents.

The reasons residents prefer to receive assistance from caregivers of the
same gender were discussed earlier in the chapter. Residents feel comfortable
when there is consistent staffing as well. It is easier to receive this type of highly
personal assistance from a few people than to have different caregivers all the
time. Because these staff members will be the most familiar with the residents
they assist, it will be easier to continually monitor and evaluate the residents'
dressing capabilities over time. These staff members will best be able to make
recommendations for individually appropriate dressing strategies.

WHAT THE ENVIRONMENT CAN DO

Designing a supportive environment to enable residents to dress more independently is critical. This section considers some environmental adaptations
that can make the bedroom more user-friendly.

Closet/Wardrobe Modification

Modifying the closet layout can help residents with dementia to make a series
of simple, highly structured decisions while dressing. As indicated in "What
Staff Can Do," residents with dementia may have trouble making decisions

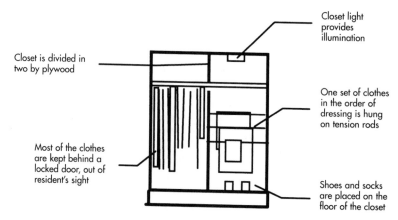

Closet light provides illumination

Closet is divided in two by plywood

One set of clothes in the order of dressing is hung on tension rods

Most of the clothes are kept behind a locked door, out of resident's sight

Shoes and socks are placed on the floor of the closet

Figure 6.3.   Modifications to closet/wardrobe that can be made that help residents with dementia in the task of dressing.

among a number of alternatives. These residents may benefit from having only a few outfits from which to select when dressing.

If the closet has two doors, then a plywood divider can be placed in the center, and a lock can be installed on one door or a hook closure added higher on the door itself (Figure 6.3). Staff can place the bulk of the residents' clothing on one side of the closet/wardrobe. On the other side, staff can place one outfit if the resident cannot make any choices, or two if he or she still enjoys having a choice. To simplify the dressing process further, install tension drapery rods over which clothing can hang. These rods should be at heights that the resident can conveniently reach and should be parallel to each other. Each rod holds one piece of clothing, with the entire outfit placed in the order in which a person normally dresses. For example, underwear can be placed on the first rod, the second rod can hold a shirt or blouse, and the third rod can have pants or a skirt. Finally, socks and shoes can be placed on the floor of the closet.

If the closet/wardrobe has only one door, an over-the-door multiple-hanger rack can be installed to display clothing (Figure 6.4). Clothes again can be placed on hangers in the order the resident would use to get dressed. If the resident has difficulties in making decisions, then the over-the-door hanger rack can be used to display only one outfit. If the resident is able to make choices when limited options are provided, then two outfits can be placed on the hanger rack. Staff can ask the resident to select from the two available options. Enabling residents to make choices promotes resident self-satisfaction and self-esteem.

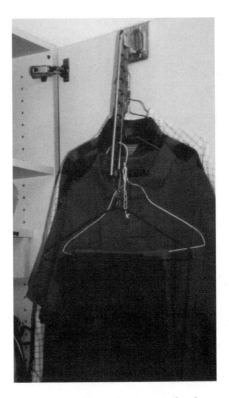

Figure 6.4. Use of an over-the-door hanger on a single-door closet to display clothing.

Selecting clothing also can be made easier by mounting an adjustable-height rod in the closet to a person's height. Tension rods easily can be added to provide two hanging levels in most closets. Similarly, using sliding shelves or drawers can help residents to reach in and get their own clothing with less staff assistance. Multiple kinds of closet systems are available that can make clothing easy to reach, and some have the added benefit of making clothing more visible.

Drawer pulls and handles should be easy to manipulate even for people with limited dexterity in their hands. C-shaped handles are easier to grasp than are small knobs. Handles that are parallel to the floor also may be difficult to grasp. Residents with extremely limited dexterity may find it easier to use handles mounted at a 45° angle to the floor. This position permits easier grasping without the person turning the wrist. Drawers should open and close smoothly without sticking. Regularly oiling all rollers and glides maximizes the operation of these items. If residents are using their own furniture and it has wooden glides, then make sure the glide surfaces are free of dirt and are soaped for lubrication. Roller glides make opening drawers easier for residents who are frail. Consider installing roller glides on larger drawers in particular for easy operation.

Recognizing the Contents of Closets

Residents with dementia, low vision, or both may have trouble recognizing or remembering where specific clothing is located behind solid doors and drawer fronts. A low-cost solution to consider is to label drawers with signs in a large typeface describing the contents of each drawer. Lettering should be at least 1 inch tall. For residents who are able to read, staff can point out these signs when assisting them with dressing. (See "What Staff Can Do" for more detailed information.)

Open shelving or wire baskets also may make it easier for residents to see clothing. Retrofitting existing wardrobes and closets with these devices is a relatively inexpensive alteration. A number of closet systems with these storage options are available at home improvement stores. Also, staff should try to keep closet floors uncluttered so that it is easier to see what items are there as well as provide better access, less distraction, and fewer possibilities of falling.

Closet and Room Lighting

Some residents may make inappropriate clothing choices simply because they cannot see the contents of the closet well. Many of us have had the experience of getting dressed in the dark and putting on one black shoe and one brown shoe. When this happened, you probably did not think that this problem was due to dementia. Therefore, it is important to consider whether each resident's dressing problems are truly cognitive or due to poor lighting.

Few facilities provide adequate lighting in bedrooms. Often, the only light in the room comes from the light fixture over the bed. To determine whether the facility should add additional lighting in the closet and dressing areas, staff should put on a pair of dark sunglasses with the eyepieces smeared with petroleum jelly and then try to select appropriate clothing from a closet. If more light is needed, then the facility can install either a light that turns on automatically when the door is opened (Figure 6.5) or a light that needs to be turned on manually. Pressure-sensitive switches can be installed on the door frames of closets to provide automatic closet lighting similar to that in a refrigerator. The cost to provide lights in the closet/wardrobe can be prohibitive when it involves rewiring, but there are other alternatives. Facilities with limited budgets can consider using battery-powered closet lights. Battery-

AliMed, Inc.
297 High Street
Dedham, MA 02026
(800) 225-2610
www.alimed.com

AdaptAbility
75 Mill Street
Colchester, CT 06415
(800) 288-9941
www.adaptability.com

Lifestyle Fascination, Inc.
110 Lehigh Street
Lakewood, NJ 08701
(800) 669-0987
www.shoplifestyle.com

Maxi-Aids
42 Executive Boulevard
Farmingdale, NY 11735
(800) 522-6294
www.maxiaids.com

Sears Home Health
9804 Chartwell
Dallas, TX 75238
(800) 326-1750

The Safety Zone
2515 East 43rd Street
Post Office Box 182247
Chattanooga, TN 37422
(800) 999-3030
www.safetyzone.com

◆ ◆ ◆

A summary sheet follows, which condenses the chapter text into a quick overview. The authors have also provided an area for you to make your own notes about your own staff and facility. Managerial staff may wish to use the summary sheets as handouts to accompany direct care staff training, or to post them by the time clock or nurses' station or include them in staff's pay envelopes.

DRESSING SUMMARY SHEET

1. Well-being and self-esteem are often linked to personal appearance.
2. The need for assistance often affects these feelings and invades privacy and personal space.
3. Changes in mobility, increased frailty, and sensory and cognitive impairments affect residents' ability to dress.

What Staff Can Do

1. Understand residents' reactions and feelings.
2. Support privacy and assist only at the required level.
3. Evaluate dressing abilities and use the 5 Ws to determine specific problems and solutions.
4. Support individual resident clothing preferences, dressing sequences, and accessories.
5. If necessary, limit choices to a few favorite outfits.
6. Set up clothing in an accessible location and in the resident's preferred order of putting it on.
7. Break down dressing tasks into simple sequences.
8. Enlist professional help (occupational therapist/physical therapist) in evaluating dressing difficulties.
9. Encourage comfortable clothing and shoes, especially for residents who use wheelchairs.
10. Provide consistent, same-sex caregivers if possible.

What the Environment Can Do

1. Divide closets to offer limited clothing choices and/or to present clothing in sequence. These closets can store/offer clothing at a variety of heights.
2. Provide good drawer pulls and glides that are maintained well.
3. Label drawers and/or provide open wire baskets.
4. Provide a dressing/grooming area with a seat and mirror, privacy, and good lighting.
5. Provide both auditory and visual privacy.
6. Install lights in closets or in places that provide adequate illumination for residents to select clothing.
7. Use adjustable closet rods that can be lowered for short people or those in wheelchairs.
8. Provide places for people to sit while dressing.

YOUR NOTES

7
Bathing

Bathing is another activity of daily living (ADL) with which many long-term care residents need assistance as their cognitive and physical abilities decline. Whereas bathing is a pleasant experience for many of us, it is often an unpleasant experience for residents of long-term care facilities as a result of both physical and mental discomfort. However, there are a number of things that can be done to make the experience more pleasant for both residents and staff.

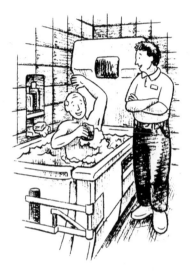

HOW IMPORTANT IS BATHING?

Bathing is something that is routine; in fact many of us do it daily. It is important to consider why we bathe, and how often it is necessary. There are three main reasons to bathe regularly: infection control, social acceptability, and pleasure. Promoting cleanliness traditionally has been a major part of nursing care. In the early 20th century, infection control also was recognized as an important reason for frequent bathing (Hektor & Touhy, 1997). As the century progressed, frequent bathing became a social norm in the United States. In fact, the idea of bathing as a way to relieve stress and pamper yourself grew so popular that many bath-related products are now sold that advertise the pleasure of bathing.

Despite all of the positive benefits associated with bathing, a number of aging-related issues may make bathing uncomfortable for residents. Older skin is more fragile and must be handled gently (e.g., patted rather than rubbed dry during personal care). Some evidence suggests that tub bathing further removes protective oils from residents' skin (Skewes, 1997). Limiting bathing to what is necessary for good hygiene and using milder soaps and lotions may help ease the dry skin and itching to which older residents are prone. A gentler skin care routine also may help prevent both skin breakdown and the incidence of pressure ulcers. (For more information about how skin changes with advancing age, see Volume 1, Chapter 5.)

WHY DO SOME RESIDENTS DISLIKE BATHING?

Memory impairments can affect a resident's feelings about bathing. Residents may think they had a bath just the day before. Today's long-term care residents come from a generation in which some people were used to bathing only once a week or only taking sink or basin baths. These may be bathing patterns they abandoned at some time during their lives, but because of the effects of dementia, they may remember only the distant past. Freeman (1997) described how bathing practices differ cross-culturally, which may be useful information in a facility with many residents who have immigrated to the United States from other countries.

Residents also may associate being cold or in pain with taking a bath. Some may recall feeling cold as they waited for the tub to fill up. Other residents with conditions such as arthritis may remember feeling pain when they were assisted in and out of a tub or shower chair. Some residents may feel that having staff assist them with bathing is an invasion of their privacy. They may be uncomfortable with staff seeing them undressed, and may think they are capable of washing themselves adequately in their own room.

HOW OFTEN SHOULD RESIDENTS BATHE?

Although many long-term care residents no longer gain pleasure from bathing, not bathing can result in skin infections and offensive odors. Staff need to consider how often each individual resident needs to bathe; for example, continent residents probably need to bathe less often than incontinent residents. Then, in instances when a resident is strongly resistant to taking a bath, staff can decide whether it is acceptable for the resident to skip or delay the bath, or they can try another method such as a giving a sink bath. Another consideration is to try to help residents regain pleasure in bathing. Ideas are offered under "What Staff Can Do" and "What the Environment Can Do."

WHAT STAFF CAN DO

Caregiving staff in long-term care facilities often are given instruction only on safety guidelines and the mechanics of bathing residents with the available equipment in the facility. Although this training is important, it is also important that staff be instructed to be aware of the residents' feelings toward bathing and of what they can do to make it a more pleasurable experience for the residents and themselves. This section includes a number of suggestions for ways that staff can ease a resident's anxiety about bathing or discomfort while bathing. Some of the recommendations mentioned here are from "Bathing Persons with Dementia" (Sloane et al., 1995). Staff should consider all of these recommendations, but bathing practices should be tailored to each resident's preferences and abilities.

Prevention of infection and odors and increased cleanliness are the obvious results that one expects from bathing. There are a number of ways of achieving these results:

- Baths (in traditional or institutional bathtub)
- Showers (standing or in a shower chair)
- Bed baths
- Sink baths
- Towel baths
- Comfort Bath or Bag Bath

The towel bath method involves washing a resident while he or she is lying in bed (Foltz-Gray, 1995; Sloane et al., 1995). A large towel and two washcloths are placed in a plastic bag with 2 quarts of warm water and 1 ounce of no-rinse soap. The water and soap are then worked into the towel and washcloths until they are damp. To bathe the resident, one part of the body is exposed, the towel is placed on the resident, and the staff member massages the skin through the towel. As other parts of the body are washed, a bath blanket should be placed on the areas already cleaned for warmth and privacy. One washcloth should be used for the face and another for the perineal (genital and anal) area. The article by Sloane et al. (1995) gives a detailed description of the step by step process. (In addition, Sloane and colleagues produced a video that shows staff the proper way to give a bath. See "Where to Find Products" for more information.)

Other forms of bathing may work better with certain residents. Comfort Bath and Bag Bath, prepackaged, disposable bathing systems that were created to be alternatives to traditional bathing, are rinse-free products that can be used for bed or seated baths. Both products come in a pouch that contains premoistened washcloths that are used to cleanse different parts of the body to reduce or eliminate cross-contamination of nonresident bacteria. The pouch contains a quick-drying cleansing solution that prevents the need for towel drying. The advantages of this system are that it is fast (5–8 minutes), replaces a traditional tub bath for maintaining good hygiene, and does not pose a problem for delicate older skin. The pouch can be heated in a warmer or microwaved briefly to warm the washcloths, and resealing the pouch keeps the rest of the washcloths warm (the Comfort Bath pouch is insulated for this purpose). (See "Where to Find Products" at the end of this chapter for sources.)

Undressing Residents

Staff should allow plenty of time for residents to do all of the steps of undressing that they still can do for themselves. This enables them both to use their remaining abilities and to feel more independent and in control. This strategy often helps to minimize combative behaviors. Some residents may not like bath time because they do not wish to get undressed for fear of becoming cold. Other residents may feel that undressing in front of someone else is an invasion of privacy. Although some loss of privacy is inevitable when assisting residents with bathing, measures can be taken to reduce these problems. Facilities with a central or shared tub room can allow high-functioning residents to choose whether to undress in the tub room or change into a robe in their bedrooms. Staff must avoid undressing residents in their rooms, simply draping them in a towel or sheet, and taking them down the hallway to the tub room.

Privacy

Because dressing is a private activity, modifications to the environment should be made for privacy. Many residents must share a room with a roommate, so it may be more appropriate to allow a resident to dress in the tub room. Robe hooks and a clothing storage area should be provided in the tub room, and a bench or chair on which a resident can sit while dressing can be considered. Make the resident bathroom a dressing area if the tub room space is limited. If a resident lives in a private room, make sure that the curtains or doors are closed to preserve the resident's privacy.

In many long-term care facilities, tub rooms either have multiple tubs or showers or are used for storing supplies or linens, so it is common for someone else to enter the room when residents are bathing. This is another invasion of privacy that can make bathing an unpleasant experience for residents and can make them resistant or combative. Develop and enforce a policy of not allowing anyone to enter the tub room when residents are being bathed. For residents who repeatedly and forcefully refuse to undress, it is sometimes easier to give a sponge bath by undressing one part of the body (such as an arm), washing it, and redressing it before moving on (Figure 7.1). In this way, residents are never completely undressed and may feel less compromised. It also may help to give residents incentives to bathe, such as promising they can have a special treat after they have bathed (e.g., a walk outside, a cup of hot tea or cocoa, a piece of chocolate).

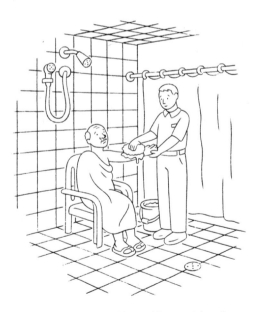

Figure 7.1. To provide residents with privacy during bathing, try draping the resident with a towel and bathing one part of the body at a time.

Running Water

Some residents can become upset or frightened by the noise or feel of water running into the tub as it fills. Most of us are used to running water into the tub before we get in and bathe. Although some institutional tubs do not allow for this, when possible, staff should fill the tub before the resident gets into it. This also can help prevent residents from becoming cold while the tub fills.

Allow residents to make choices and do tasks for themselves. Offer residents the opportunity to test the water so that they take a bath or shower at a temperature with which they are comfortable. Give residents a soapy washcloth to wash their arms while you clean the harder-to-reach areas. A large, easy-to-grip hand-held shower wand helps residents to wash themselves more easily.

Air and Water Temperatures

Residents often complain of feeling cold when they bathe, and a number of things can be done to alleviate this. First, the tub room should be kept at a temperature that is comfortable for people who are undressed. If you are unsure whether the tub room is warm enough, test it by having one staff member give another a bath. (This is also an excellent sensitivity training experience.) Place towels or blankets over the shoulders or laps of residents who say that they are cold. Wet hair easily can make a person cold; therefore, hair should be washed at the end of the bath and the resident's head wrapped with a towel immediately after the hair is washed.

WHAT THE ENVIRONMENT CAN DO

The environment plays a key role in the bathing experience. Tub rooms in most long-term care facilities usually are unfamiliar places that frequently confuse and agitate residents. It may be difficult for residents with dementia to bathe themselves because of impaired physical and cognitive abilities or complicated tubs. The following suggestions will help to make bathing a more positive experience.

Using a Tub that Fits Residents' Needs

When planning to buy new bathing tubs, facilities should consider the options offered by different models (Table 7.1). A tub that can be filled before the resident enters it is best for high-functioning residents. This type of tub is more

Table 7.1. Comparison of bathing tub models

	Side-entry tilting tubs	Front-entry tubs	Side-entry tubs with door	Lift-over tubs
Use	Lift-up side doors and a pre-filled water footwell; once resident has entered the tub, tub tilts back and water from the footwell fills remainder of tub	Front-entry door that works well with special chairs or lifts that glide resident back into bathing areas; prefilled chamber fills tub with temperature-adjusted water in 90 seconds after door is shut	Side-entry doors with built-in seats; doors may swing out, roll down or swing up, depending on model; tub fills with temperature-adjusted water after door is shut	These tubs require a resident be lifted over to enter it; tub can be raised or lowered to aid the caregiver
Options and features	Companion lifts Adjustable heights Remote locatable controls Electric tilt Hand-held shower wand	Companion carrier Available with UV light (eliminates bacteria) Hand-held shower wands	Companion lifts Can be mounted in a recess similar to a residential tub Hand-held shower wands	Companion lifts Some models can be raised and lowered
Pros	Emulates actual bathing by allowing bather to adjust to water temperature before being immersed in water Controls can be located behind a curtain to lessen institutional appearance Side entry allows for easy transfer of ambulatory residents Whole body of resident easily reachable by caregiver	Offers quick bathing with 90-second fill and quick drain Tub temperature and water level controlled by the tub once set rather than staff monitoring Tub allows for fairly easy transfer of nonambulatory residents into tub	With built-in appearance on some models it can resemble a residential tub Side-entry door provides dignified entry for ambulatory residents Some models allow for resident to bathe unassisted	Some units allow supine bathing Can use a standard residential tub in a recessed platform for a residential appearance

continued

173

Table 7.1. *continued*

	Side-entry tilting tubs	Front-entry tubs	Side-entry tubs with door	Lift-over tubs
Cons	Tilting of tub may disorient some residents Tub has an institutional appearance Motion of some manual hydraulic models may be jerky Because of how it operates, tub must be used with assistance	Quick water fill from behind may disturb some residents Tub has an institutional appearance Some residents may not like cold room temperature while waiting for tub to fill Ambulatory residents still must use transfer chair and be assisted when bathing Feet of resident are positioned low and hard to reach	Nonresidential controls may confuse/disturb residents Some seats are too upright and use straps to keep residents from slouching Some large doors are difficult to operate and may pinch residents Some residents may not like cold room temperature while waiting for tub to fill	Lift-over chairs can be frightening for resident and difficult for staff to use Companion lifts are only way to easily transfer a resident who is unable to step over tub Low tubs may be difficult for caregiver to use Some models can be very institutional in appearance
Sources	Arjo, Inc. 50 N. Gary Avenue Roselle, IL 60172 (800) 323-1245 *www.arjo.com*	Apollo P.O. Box 219 450 Main Street Somerset, WI 54025 (800) 247-5490 (715) 247-5625 *www.apollobath.com*	Apollo P.O. Box 219 450 Main Street Somerset, WI 54025 (800) 247-5490 (715) 247-5625 *www.apollobath.com* Arjo, Inc. 50 N. Gary Avenue Roselle, IL 60172 (800) 323-1245 *www.arjo.com* Invacare 739 Goddard Avenue Chesterfield, MO 63005 (800) 347-5440 *www.invacare-ccg.com*	Arjo, Inc. 50 N. Gary Avenue Roselle, IL 60172 (800) 323-1245 *www.arjo.com* Invacare 739 Goddard Avenue Chesterfield, MO 63005 (800) 347-5440 *www.invacare-ccg.com*

familiar, and residents can test the water temperature before bathing. Staff can explain to residents what is about to happen before they are immersed in the water. It is also best to avoid purchasing tubs that require lifting the resident in a chair over the side of the tub. This can be a frightening experience for residents because it is not familiar to them. Several tub models can be filled first and do not require a chair lift (see "Where to Find Products").

Facilities that have a relatively high percentage of residents with significant impairments should consider buying a tub that accommodates both seated and supine bathing. Several models do not require the resident to be lifted high off the ground, and therefore may be less frightening to residents with dementia. Some older facilities may have large institutional floor-mounted tubs that resemble standard residential tubs. These tubs are difficult for staff and residents to use. Slide transfer benches can make these tubs more usable for staff (see "Where to Find Products" for sources).

Some residents may dislike showers because they do not have control over the stream of water hitting them. For example, depending on their height, or if they are sitting on a shower chair, the stream of water may hit them in the face or make their hair wet. The facility should consider installing hand-held shower wands so that staff can control where the water flows. Some residents may be able to hold and direct these showerheads themselves. Most showerheads can be retrofitted easily at little expense. Showerheads with wands also should have a holder that slides on a vertical bar. This bar allows the shower wand to be mounted at different heights. The installation kit should give instructions about where the bar should be placed to take advantage of these features.

Privacy Issues

Several privacy issues and solutions were discussed under "What Staff Can Do." Facilities that are planning to remodel their tub rooms can make environmental modifications to provide privacy. One modification is to partition the room in such a way as to make private bathing compartments with actual doors. Privacy in shower areas also should be considered. A half-height shower curtain that hooks across the shower opening provides some privacy for residents and keeps the staff dry (see "Where to Find Products"). However, these curtains are not a substitute for privacy curtains.

Controlling Air and Water Temperatures

Tub rooms can feel cold to an undressed resident, particularly if the temperature cannot be individually controlled. If a resident indicates that he or

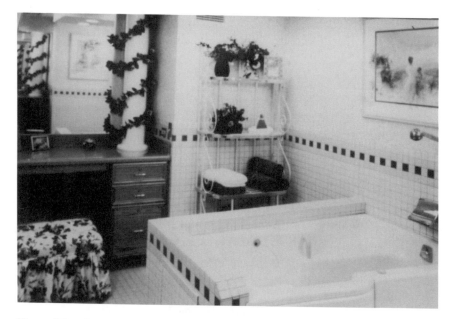

Figure 7.2.   Certain decor in the tub room may remind residents of home.

she is cold, then bathing the resident under a sheet or covering him or her with a soft towel may reduce agitation. (This was explained in more detail under "What Staff Can Do.") Facilities with consistently cold tub rooms should consider installing a heat lamp or a radiant heat panel (see "Where to Find Products").

Creating Pleasant Tub Rooms

Seldom in long-term care is attention paid to making bathing a pleasurable experience. In addition to the interventions mentioned in "What Staff Can Do," several environmental modifications can make bathing more pleasurable, or at least less upsetting. For example, decorating the bathroom so that it is visually interesting makes it appear less institutional and can provide distractions (Figure 7.2). Decorations that are moisture resistant or plasticized hold up longer. Decorative curtains for the windows, around the tub, or even below the sink can add a homelike touch. A number of plants that like a moist atmosphere can thrive in a bathroom (see Volume 4, Appendix C, for a list of nontoxic plants), although grow lights may be necessary if the bathroom has no windows. Painting the room a warm peach or coral can make the tub room feel warmer even though it will not actually change the temperature of the tub room. These colors also flatter skin tones and as a result may make the bathing experience more pleasant for residents. Avoid using cooler paint colors or shades that do not flatter skin tones in these rooms. Improper color choice can make residents look sick or jaundiced.

Try to create a grooming area with a vanity, seat, and mirror. This might be as easy as providing a skirted table with a mirror hung above it. A large flower arrangement or old perfume and lotion bottles placed on the vanity can make the room seem more homelike. Providing a place for residents to keep clothes that they can put on after bathing will be appreciated by many residents.

Staff can determine the resident's favorite soothing music and play it when the resident enters the tub room. However, a little volume goes a long way in rooms with predominantly hard surfaces. Carefully monitor the volume and impact of music on the resident. Consider ways to make the room smell nice as well. Aromatherapy oils can be placed in a diffuser or on a light bulb, or a little air freshener can be sprayed around the room just before the resident enters.

Tub rooms are among the noisiest rooms in a long-term care facility, particularly when a whirlpool tub is running. Several companies make moisture-proof acoustical panels to reduce some of the noise in these rooms. These panels can be adhered to ceilings or walls that are located away from the splash zone. (See "Where to Find Products" for sources for acoustical treatments for tub rooms.)

WHERE TO FIND PRODUCTS

Videos

Solving Bathing Problems in Persons with Alzheimer's Disease and Related Dementias
Produced by Philip Sloane, M.D., M.Ph., Ann Louise Barrick, Ph.D., and Vanessa Honn
Available from Health Professions Press, (888) 337-8808, *www.health-propress.com*
Analyzes real-life bathing situations to demonstrate how flexibility, sensitivity, and persuasion can be employed to reduce aggression and agitation.

Alternative Bathing Products

Incline Technologies
(800) 538-0205
www.inclinetechnologies.com
Manufactures Bag Bath, a prepackaged disposable bathing system; moistened cloths containing a quick-evaporating cleansing solution

Sage Products, Inc.
815 Tek Drive
Post Office Box 9693
Crystal Lake, IL 60014-9693
(800) 323-2220
www.sageproducts.com
Manufactures Comfort Bath, a prepackaged system of eight disposable washcloths that can be heated in a microwave

Tubs and Showers

The following manufacturers stock a variety of tubs and showers:

Apollo Corporation
Post Office Box 219
450 Main Street
Somerset, WI 54025
(800) 247-5490
(715) 247-5625
www.apollobath.com

Aquarius Bathware LLC
Praxis Industries, Inc.
435 Industrial Road
Savannah, TN 38372
(800) 443-7269
www.aquariusproducts.com
Tub with extra-large grab bars

Arjo, Inc.
50 North Gary Avenue, Unit A
Roselle, IL 60172
(800) 323-1245
www.arjo.com
Manufactures the Parker tub

BathEase
3815 Darston Street
Palm Harbor, FL 34658
(727) 786-2604

Comfort Designs
Box 34279
Richmond, VA 23234
(800) 801-2820

Edison Lyle
Post Office Box 728
Jonesboro, GA 30237
(800) 444-0888
Manufactures Freedom Bath

Invacare
739 Goddard Avenue
Chesterfield, MO 63005
(800) 347-5440
www.invacare-ccg.com

Sunrise Medical
5001 Joerns Drive
Stevens Point, WI 54481
(800) 826-0270
www.sunrisemedical.com

Slide Transfer Benches

Clever Solutions, Inc.
2122 Agin Court
Ann Arbor, MI 48103
(734) 668-2524
Manufactures a rotating sliding transfer bench

Eagle Health Supplies
2165 North Glassell Street
Orange, CA 92865
(800) 755-8999
www.eaglehealth.com

Half-Height Shower Curtains

Invacare
739 Goddard Avenue
Chesterfield, MO 63005
(800) 347-5440
www.invacare-ccg.com
Invacare manufactures a low-hanging shower curtain for sit-down shower cabinet that provides privacy and protects those giving a bath.

Heat Lamps

Nu-Tone
Madison and Red Bank Roads
Cincinnati, OH 45227-1599
(800) 543-8687

Acoustical Treatments

Conwed Designscape
800 Gustafson Road
Ladysmith, WI 54848
(800) 932-2383
www.conweddesignscape.com

Illbruck Architectural Products
3800 Washington Avenue North
Minneapolis, MN 55412
(800) 225-1920
www.illbruck-archprod.com
Manufactures acoustical panels with stain-resistant surfaces

JM Lynne Co., Inc.
59 Gilpin Avenue
Post Office Box 1010
Smithtown, NY 11787
(800) 645-5044
www.jmlynne.com
Manufactures flame-retardant acoustical textile wallcoverings

Pyrok, Inc.
121 Sunset Road
Mamaroneck, NY 10543
(914) 777-7070
www.pyrokinc.com

◆ ◆ ◆

A summary sheet follows, which condenses the chapter text into a quick overview. The authors have also provided an area for you to make your own notes about your own staff and facility. Managerial staff may wish to use the summary sheets as handouts to accompany direct care staff training, or to post them by the time clock or nurses' station or include them in staff's pay envelopes.

BATHING SUMMARY SHEET

1. There are three key reasons for bathing: infection control, social acceptability, and pleasure/stress relief.
2. Residents may resist bathing because it is no longer pleasurable or is uncomfortable, cold, or painful. Bathing may cause dry skin and itching. The institutional bath setting is usually too dark or too bright, unfamiliar, or even frightening. Residents may have different cultural or individual ways of cleaning. Staff assistance is often perceived as an invasion of privacy.
3. The real issues may be how frequently bathing is needed and what methods are acceptable.

What Staff Can Do

1. Provide bathing alternatives: traditional or institutional tub, shower, bed bath, sink bath, or towel bath.
2. Provide privacy and dignity by ensuring adequate time to undress, wash, and dress as independently as possible.
3. Provide robes and towels to keep residents covered and as warm as possible.
4. Do not allow anyone else to enter the bathing area.
5. Try a sponge bath, washing only one uncovered part of the body at a time.
6. Before the resident gets in or is helped into the tub, fill the tub and turn off the water. Use a bath thermometer to check the water temperature, then ask the resident to test it.
7. Encourage residents to wash themselves. Use verbal cueing or demonstrate on yourself.
8. Keep the room warm enough for the comfort of a wet, naked person. Put towels or blankets over exposed body parts and hair.
9. Explore alternate methods of bathing.
10. Try very soft, soothing music according to resident preferences, and use aromatic oils.

What the Environment Can Do

1. Select the appropriate tub based on user population when remodeling.
2. Install hand-held shower wands on an adjustable-height vertical rod holder.
3. Include heat lamps or radiant heat panels to warm rooms, especially during seasons when the facility's heat is not turned on.
4. Subdivide large spaces to make bathing scale more residential.
5. Use attractive, residential-style window, shower, and privacy curtains.
6. Decorate in ways that are both attractive and visually interesting to provide residents with both a comfortable atmosphere and distractions.

7. Create a dressing area with vanity, seat, and mirror.
8. Reduce frightening or annoying noise levels by using moisture-proof acoustic panels.

YOUR NOTES

Bibliography

Americans with Disabilities Act (ADA) of 1990, PL 101-336, 42 U.S.C. §§ 12101 *et seq.*

Andresen, G. (1995). *Caring for people with Alzheimer's disease: A training manual for direct care providers.* Baltimore: Health Professions Press.

Baker, S.P., O'Neill, B., Ginsburg, M.J., & Guohua, L. (1992). *The injury fact book* (2nd ed.). New York: Oxford University Press.

Baucom, A.H. (1996). *Hospitality design for the graying generation.* New York: John Wiley & Sons.

Bayles, K., & Tomoeda, C. (1995). *The ABC's of dementia.* Tucson, AZ: Canyonlands Publishing.

Beck, C. (1988). Measurement of dressing performance in persons with dementia. *American Journal of Alzheimer's Care and Related Disorders & Research, 3*(3), 21–25.

Birren, J., & Schaie, K. (1990). *Handbook of the psychology of aging* (3rd ed.). San Diego: Harcourt, Brace, Jovanovich.

Bowlby, C. (1993). *Therapeutic activities with persons disabled by Alzheimer's disease and related disorders.* Gaithersburg, MD: Aspen Publishers.

Braun, J., & Lipson, S. (1993). *Toward a restraint free environment: Reducing the use of physical and chemical restraints in long-term and acute care settings.* Baltimore: Health Professions Press.

Brawley, E.C. (1997). *Designing for Alzheimer's disease: Strategies for creating better care environments.* New York: John Wiley & Sons.

Brush, J.A., & Camp, C.J. (1998). *A therapy technique for improving memory: Spaced retrieval.* Beechwood, OH: Menorah Park Center for Aging.

Burns, R., Moskowitz, M., Ash, A., Kane, R., Finch, M., & McCarthy, E. (1997). Variations in the performance of hip fracture procedures. *Medical Care, 35*(3), 196–203.

Calkins, M.P. (1988). *Design for dementia: Planning environments for the elderly and the confused.* Owings Mills, MD: National Health Publishing.

Calkins, M.P (1989). Design strategies to curb unsafe walking. *Provider, 15*(8), 7, 10.

Carpman, J.R. (1991). Wayfinding in health care: 6 common myths. *Health Facilities Management, 4*(5), 24–28.

Carpman, J.R., Grant, M., & Simmons, D. (1985). *No more mazes: Research about design and wayfinding in hospitals.* Ann Arbor: University of Michigan Press.

Chandler, J.M., & Duncan, P.W. (1993). Balance and falls in the elderly: Issues in evaluation and treatment. In Guccione, A. (Ed.), *Geriatric physical therapy* (pp. 237–251). St. Louis: Mosby/YearBook.

Cohen, U., & Weisman, G. (1991). *Holding on to home.* Baltimore: The Johns Hopkins University Press.

Denney, A. (1997). Quiet music: An intervention for mealtime agitation? *Journal of Gerontological Nursing, 23*(7), 16–23.

Dube, A., & Mitchell, E. (1986). Accidental strangulation from vest restraints. *Journal of the American Medical Association, 256*(19), 2725–2726.

Eliopoulos, C. (2000). *Gerontological nursing* (5th ed.). Philadelphia: Lippincott Williams & Wilkins.

Emlet, C.A., Crabtree, J.L., Condon, V.A., & Treml, L.A. (1996). *In-home assessment of older adults: An interdisciplinary approach.* Gaithersburg, MD: Aspen Publishers.

Epstein, B. (1994). Wandering and liability revisited. *Provider, 20*(12), 29.

Evans, L.K. (1987). Sundown syndrome in institutionalized elderly. *Journal of the American Geronotological Society, 35,* 101–108.

Evans, L.K. (1991). Nursing care and management of behavioral problems in the elderly. In M.S. Harper (Ed.), *Management and care of the elderly: Psychosocial perspectives* (pp. 191–206). Newbury Park, CA: Sage Publications.

Foltz-Gray, D. (1995). Rough waters. *Contemporary Long-Term Care, 18*(9), 66–70.

Freeman, E.M. (1997). International perspectives on bathing. *Journal of Gerontological Nursing, 23*(5), 40–44.

Gallo, J., Reichel, W., & Andersen, L. (Eds.). (1995). *Handbook of geriatric assessment* (2nd ed.). Gaithersburg, MD: Aspen Publishers.

Genevay, B. (1997). See me! Hear me! Know who I am! An experience of being assessed: The client's perspective. *Generations, 21*(1), 16–18.

Gray-Micelli, D.L., Waxman, H., Cavalieri, T., & Lage, S. (1994). Prodromal falls among older nursing home residents. *Applied Nursing Research, 7,* 18–27.

Guccione, A.A. (1993). Functional assessment of the elderly. In A.A. Guccione (Ed.), *Geriatric physical therapy* (pp. 113–123). St. Louis: Mosby/YearBook.

Hall, G.R. (1994, April). Chronic dementia: Challenges in feeding a patient. *Journal of Gerontological Nursing,* 21–30.

Hall, G., & Buckwalter, K. (1987). Progressively lowered stress threshold: A conceptual model for care of adults with Alzheimer's disease. *Archives of Psychiatric Nursing, 1*(6), 399–406.

Hektor, L., & Touhy, T. (1997). The history of the bath: From art to task? Reflections for the future. *Journal of Gerontological Nursing, 23*(5), 7–18.

Hellen, C. (1990). Eating: An Alzheimer activity. *American Journal of Alzheimer's Care and Related Disorders & Research, 5*(2), 5–9.

Hiatt, L. (1991). *Nursing home renovation designed for reform.* Boston: Butterworth Architecture.

Illuminating Engineering Society of North America. (1998). *Lighting and the visual environment for senior living* (RP-28-98). New York: IESNA.

Johnson, D. (1995). Restraint-free care. *Nursing Homes, 44*(8), 26–30.

Kane, R.A., & Kane, R.L. (1981). *Assessing the elderly: A practical guide to measurement.* Lexington, MA: Lexington Books.

Kovach, C., Weisman, G., Choudhury, H., & Calkins, M. (1997). Impacts of a therapeutic environment on dementia care. *American Journal of Alzheimer's Disease & Related Disorders, 12*(3), 99–109.

Lawton, M.P., Fulcomer, M., & Kleban, M. (1984). Architecture for the mentally impaired elderly. *Environment and Behavior, 16*(6), 730–757.

Lawton, M.P., & Nahemow, L. (1973). Ecology and the aging process. In C. Eisdorfer & M.P. Lawton (Eds.), *Psychology of adult development and aging.* Washington, DC: American Psychological Association.

Leibowitz, B., Lawton, M.P., & Waldman, A. (1979). Evaluation: Designing for confused elderly patients. *American Institute of Architects Journal, 68,* 59–61.

Mace, N., & Rabins, P.V. (1981). *The 36-hour day.* Baltimore: The Johns Hopkins University Press.

McGuineas, W.J., Stein, B., & Reynolds, J.S. (1980). Mechanical and electrical equipment for buildings. New York: John Wiley & Sons.

Moody, H. (1992). *Ethics in an aging society.* Baltimore: The Johns Hopkins University Press.

Morse, J.M., Tylko, S.J., & Dixon, H.A. (1987). Characteristics of the fall-prone patient. *Gerontologist, 27,* 516–522.

Namazi, K.H. (1990). *Effect of personalized cues at bedrooms on wayfinding among institutionalized elders with Alzheimer's disease.* Paper presented at the American Psychological Association annual meeting, Boston.

Namazi, K.H., & Johnson, B.D. (1991a). Environmental effects on incontinence problems in Alzheimer's disease patients. *American Journal of Alzheimer's Care and Related Disorders & Research, 6*(6), 16–21.

Namazi, K.H., & Johnson, B.D. (1991b). Physical environmental cues to reduce the problems of incontinence in Alzheimer disease units. *American Journal of Alzheimer's Care and Related Disorders & Research, 6,* 22–28.

Namazi, K.H., & Johnson, B.D. (1992a). Dressing independently: A closet modification model for Alzheimer's disease patients. *American Journal of Alzheimer's Care and Related Disorders & Research, 7*(1), 16–28.

Namazi, K.H., & Johnson, B.D. (1992b). Environmental issues related to visibility and consumption of food in an Alzheimer's disease unit. *American Journal of Alzheimer's Care and Related Disorders & Research, 7,* 30–34.

Namazi, K.H., Rosner, T.T., & Rechlin, L.R. (1991).Long-term memory cueing to reduce visuo-spatial disorientation in Alzheimer's disease patients in a special care unit. *American Journal of Alzheimer's Care and Related Disorders & Research, 6*(6), 10–15.

Omnibus Budget Reconciliation Act of 1987, PL. No. 100-203, § 2, 101 Stat. 1330 (1987).

Ostasz, J. (1986). Successful techniques for hand-feeding the elderly. *Geriatric Care, 18*(11), 1–4.

Passini, R., & Proulx, G. (1988). Wayfinding without vision: An experiment with congenitally totally blind people. *Environment and Behavior, 20*(2), 227–252.

Payten, A., & Porter, V. (1994). Armchair aerobics for the cognitively impaired. *Activities, Adaptation, and Aging, 18*(2), 27–37.

Rader, J., Doan, J., & Schwab, M. (1985). How to decrease wandering: A form of agenda behavior. *Geriatric Nursing, 6*(4), 196–199.

Rush, K.L., & Ouellet, L.L. (1997). Mobility aids and the elderly client. *Journal of Gerontological Nursing, 7–15.*

Skewes, S.M. (1997). Bathing: It's a tough job! *Journal of Gerontological Nursing, 23*(5), 45–49.

Sloane, P., Rader, J., Barrick, A., Hoeffer, B., Dwyer, S., McKenzie, D., Lavelle, M., Buckwalter, K., Arrington, L., & Pruitt, T. (1995). Bathing persons with dementia. *Gerontologist, 35,* 672–678.

Soltesz, K.S., & Dayton, J.H. (1995, November/December). The effects of menu modification to increase dietary intake and maintain the weight of Alzheimer residents. *American Journal of Alzheimer's Disease,* 20–23.

Tappen, R.M., Roach, K.E., Buchner, D., Barry, C., & Edelstein, J. (1997). Reliability of physical performance measures in nursing home residents with Alzheimer's disease. *Journal of Gerontology, 52A*(1), M52–M55.

Teresi, J., Lawten, M., Holmes, D., & Ory, M. (1997). *Measurement in elderly chronic care populations.* New York: Springer Publishing.

Thomas, W. (1996). *Life worth living.* Acton, MA: Wanderwyk & Burnham.

Tideiksaar, R. (1998). *Falls in older persons: Prevention & management* (2nd ed.). Baltimore: Health Professions Press.

Treml, L. (1996). Basic mobility needs. In C.E.A. Emlet (Ed.), *In home assessment of older adults: An interdisciplinary approach* (pp. 50–75). Gaithersburg, MD: Aspen Publishers.

Verfaillie, D., Nichols, J., Turkel, E., & Havell, M. (1997). Effects of resistance, balance, and gait training on reduction of risk factors leading to falls in elders. *Journal of Aging and Physical Activity, 5,* 213–228.

Volicer, L., Seltzer, B., Rheaume, Y., Karner, J., Glennon, M., Riley, M., & Crino, P. (1989). Eating difficulties in patients with probable dementia of the Alzheimer type. *Journal of Geriatric Psychiatry and Neurology, 2*(4), 188–195.

Wise, K. (1996, July/August). Making the choice to carpet. *Nursing Homes,* 17–20.

Wykle, M.L. (1993). An overview of restraint use and the movement to reduce the use of restraints. In J. Braun & S. Lipson (Eds.), *Toward a restraint-free environment: Reducing the use of physical and chemical restraints in long-term care and acute care settings* (pp. 3–10). Baltimore: Health Professions Press.

Zavotka, S.L., & Teaford, M.H. (1997). The design of shared social spaces in assisted living residences for older adults. *Journal of Interior Design, 23*(2), 2–16.

Zgola, J.M., & Bordillon, G. (2001). *Bon appetit! The joy of dining in long-term care.* Baltimore: Health Professions Press.

Index

Page numbers followed by *f* indicate figures; those followed by *t* indicate tables. This is a comprehensive index covering Volumes 1–4 of *Creating Successful Dementia Care Settings*. The first number of each entry indicates the volume; the second number indicates the page.

Acoustical treatments, 2.180, 3.100
  for bathing, 2.177, 2.180
  dining room ceilings, 2.130
  and excess background noise,
    1.29–1.30, 3.95
  walls, 2.139
Activities
  appropriate, providing, 4.49–4.54, 4.57
    encouraging participation, 4.57
    ensuring success, 4.54–4.56
    identifying from life areas, 4.51–4.54
    and reality orientation, 4.56
  domestic-based, 4.52–4.53, 4.58–4.60
  leisure-based, 4.53–4.54
  limiting conflict with therapy, 2.68
  reinvolving residents, 4.48
    with impaired hearing, 1.28
    with impaired vision, 1.9–1.11
  residents' choice in, 4.107, 4.111
  and residents' life roles, *see* Roles, as
    self-definition
  work-based, 4.53
  see also History, resident's, gathering;
    specific activities
Activities of daily living (ADLs)
  and Beck Dressing Performance scale,
    2.147
  and combative behaviors, 3.80
    emotional issues, 3.83–3.84
    providing clear explanations, 3.86,
      3.104
    using routine as an intervention,
      3.84–3.85
  and functional abilities, *see* Functional
    abilities

IADLs, *see* Independent activities of
    daily living
  and mobility, *see* Mobility
  residents' preferences, considering,
    4.105–4.107
  and sensory impairments, 1.1
  see also specific ADLs
ADA, *see* Americans with Disabilities Act
    of 1990
Adaptive equipment, 2.162–2.163
Adjustable-height tables, *see* Tables,
    dining; Furniture, residential-style
ADLs, *see* Activities of daily living and
    Beck Dressing Performance scale
Affection, need for, as trigger for inap-
    propriate behavior, 3.109–3.110
Agenda behavior approach, 3.4–3.5
  behavior tracking process, 3.5–3.7
    five Ws, 3.5–3.6
    resident's history, 3.6
  and dressing, 2.151–2.152
  and wandering, *see* Wandering
Aggressive behaviors, 3.2
  and agenda behavior, 3.4
  triggers for, 3.75, 3.76
  see also Combative behaviors
Aging, myths about, 2.2–2.3
Agitation, *see* Anxiety; Combative
    behaviors
Agnosia, 2.6, 2.14
Air circulation, 1.37
Alarms
  clothing cords, 2.72
  door, 3.54–3.55
  emergency, altering, 3.49

Alarms—*continued*
    beepers, 3.93, 3.100–3.101
Americans with Disabilities Act (ADA) of
    1990 (PL 101-336), guidelines,
    1.21, 2.19–2.20, 2.31, 2.73, 2.99
Anxiety
    addressing, 3.16
    and combative behaviors, 3.79
    buildup, 3.81
    orientation and, 2.13
Aphasia, 2.6
Appetite, physical factors affecting,
    2.104–2.105, 2.105*f*, 2.106
Apraxia, 2.6, 2.49, 2.147
Aromas, as mealtime environmental
    cues, 2.35
Aromatherapy, 1.37, 1.38*f*, 3.92, 3.102,
    3.112, 4.34
Art
    hanging, 4.23, 4.34–4.35, 4.161–4.162,
        4.161*f*
    interactive, 4.33
        as diversion intervention, 3.23,
            3.24*f*, 3.29, 3.32
        as orientation device, 3.24,
            3.38–3.39
Aspiration, 2.108, 2.109
Assessment, of functional abilities, 2.7–2.8
    cognitive factors, 2.9
    environmental factors, 2.10
    physical factors, 2.8
    social factors, 2.9–2.10
Attempting to leave, 3.39–3.40
    and agenda behavior, 3.4, 3.41
    confinement, minimizing, 3.45
    and dementia, 4.15
    distraction, 3.43–3.44, 3.46, 3.48
    and negative odors, 1.36
    redirecting, 3.41, 3.42–3.43, 3.44*f*
    shadowing, 3.40
    successful exiting, staff responses to,
        3.44–3.45
    and timed activities, 3.42, 3.58–3.60
    triggers, 3.43*t*
        tracking, 3.40, 3.41*f*
    and wandering, 3.10
Autonomy, 4.93–4.94
    choice, 4.94–4.95
    and relocation, 4.99–4.100
    sacrificing, reasons for, 4.99
    well-being, 4.95–4.96
    see also Control

BASs, *see* Bed alarm systems
Bathing, 2.167–2.182
    and air temperature, 2.172, 2.180
    alternative products, 2.177–2.178, 3.97
    and combative behavior, 2.177
        appropriate bathtubs, *see* Bathtubs
        considering purpose of bath, 3.85
        hand-held shower wands, 3.88, 3.89*f*
        music and, 3.85–3.86
        natural elements and, 3.86
        preserving privacy, 3.85
        using routines to prevent, 3.84–3.85
        using texture to reduce, 1.44
        undressing, and ways to prevent,
            3.84
    disliking, reasons for, 2.167, 2.168
    frequency of, 2.168–2.169
    minimizing negative scents, 1.35–1.36
    music in, 2.177
    noise reduction, 2.177
    and positive scents, 1.34–1.35
    prepackaged bath, 2.170
    privacy, preserving, 2.170–2.171, 2.175,
        4.82–4.83, 4.84–4.85
    slide transfer benches, 2.175, 2.179
    towel bath, 2.169–2.170
    undressing for, 2.170
    water
        residents' concerns about, 2.172
        temperature, 2.172, 2.175–2.176
    see also Tub rooms
Bathrooms
    and privacy, 4.87
    private, decorating, 4.26–4.27, 4.129
    wayfinding, 2.33–2.34, 2.96
        use of canopies in, 2.34
        use of color in, 2.34
        use of signage in, 2.35*f*, 2.97*f*
        toilet, finding, 2.35, 2.96–2.97,
            2.98*f*
Bathtubs, 2.178–2.179, 3.90–3.91,
    3.98–3.99
    appropriate, 2.172, 2.173*t*–2.174*t*,
        2.175, 3.88–3.89
    models, 3.90–3.91
    see also Tub rooms
Beck Dressing Performance scale, 2.147,
    2.148
Bed alarm systems (BASs), 2.82–2.83,
    2.84
Bedrails, 2.81
    alternatives to, 2.81

Bedrooms
  arthritis, residents with, 2.81
  decor, 2.33, 2.80, 4.24–4.26,
      4.125–4.129, 4.125*f*
  decorating, 4.22–4.26
  flooring, 2.80
  furniture, 2.80–2.81, 4.86
  lighting, 2.79–2.80
  Parkinson's disease, residents with,
      2.80–2.81
  personalization, encouraging,
      4.17–4.18
  privacy
    room assignments for, 4.86
    in shared, 4.85–4.86, 4.87*f*
  wayfinding, 2.29–2.33
    decorating for, 4.27–4.28
    display cases, 2.30–2.31, 2.31*f*, 4.28,
        4.29*f*
    lighting, use of, 2.29–2.30
    window treatments, 4.28–4.29
Behavior tracking process, 3.5–3.7, 4.106
  Behavior Tracking Form, 3.6, 3.127–3.129
  see also Ws, five
Benches, slide transfer, *see* Slide transfer
    benches
Boredom, and rummaging, 3.66
"Bowling alley," 3.16–3.17, 3.17*f*
Buildup, *see* Anxiety

Cabinets, as room dividers, *see* Room
    dividers
Calcium metabolism, and light, 1.7
Call bell systems, 2.82
Call lights, 2.72
Calm perseverance, 3.111
Canes, 2.63, 2.64*t*
Cardiovascular problems, and mobility,
    2.45
Care
  models
    and autonomy, 4.100
    hospitality, 4.5–4.6
    medical, 4.2–4.3
    residential, 4.3–4.5
    and residents' life roles, 4.46–4.47
  provision, *see* Activities of daily living
  resistance to, *see* Combative behaviors
Carpeting, 2.85, 2.137–2.138,
    4.136–4.137
  for bedrooms, 4.127–4.128

  for dining areas, 2.128
  and mobility, 2.69, 2.70
  odor-resistant, 1.36
  quiet vacuum cleaners, 2.87–2.88,
      2.138–2.139
  and resilient flooring, comparison,
      2.129*t*–2.130*t*
  -to-tile transitions, 2.86
Cataracts, 1.5, 1.6*t*
  overall blurred vision, 1.6
Ceiling tiles, and excess background
    noise, 1.29–1.30
Chairs
  alarms, 2.81
  dining, 2.125–2.126, 2.125*f*,
      2.135–2.136, 4.135, 4.139–4.140;
      see also Dining rooms
  gliding/rocking, 3.29, 3.34–3.35
  and hallways, 2.20, 2.20*f*
  and mobility, 2.81
  seating arrangements for privacy,
      4.88–4.89
Challenging behaviors, *see* Disruptive
    behavior
Charts, residents'
  combative behaviors, recording, 3.80,
      4.51
  importance of documenting
      preferences, 1.31, 1.35, 1.43, 1.46,
      4.49–4.51
  see also History, residents', gathering
Childlike activities, avoiding, 4.57
Choice, exercising, 4.94–4.95
Circadian rhythms, and natural light, 1.7
Closets
  adjustable-height rods, 2.159
  dividing, 2.158
  drawers, 2.159–2.160
  lighting, 2.160–2.161, 2.161*f*
  organizing, 2.152
  racks, 2.158, 2.159*f*
Clothing, and dressing issues, *see*
    Dressing
Cluster floor plan, 2.23–2.24, 2.24*f*, 4.122
Cognitive impairment
  and sensory impairment, 1.2
  and wandering, 3.11
Color
  and appetite, 2.124
  contrast, 1.20, 2.70, 2.97, 2.132–2.133
  as orientation device, 2.25–2.26, 2.34,
      3.24, 3.25

Color—*continued*
  and pattern, *see* Pattern
  rendering, 1.13–1.14
  room paint, 2.176–2.177, 4.24–4.27,
    4.126–4.128
  in signage, 3.25
Color Rendering Index, 1.13, 1.17
Combative behaviors, 3.1, 3.2,
  3.75–3.104
  charting, *see* Charts, residents'
  frequency of, 3.76
  impact of on other residents,
    3.76–3.77
  resistance to care, 3.75–3.76, 3.80,
    3.81*f*, 4.79–4.80
  and restraints, 3.3, 3.81–3.82
  staff responses to, 3.77
    intervening, 3.87–3.88
    training, 3.82–3.83
    tracking, 3.80
  triggers for, 3.77–3.79
    agitation as a precursor, 3.82
  see also specific ADLs
Common areas
  arrangement of, 1.22
    for privacy, 4.88–4.89, 4.90*f*
  decorating, 4.29–4.31, 4.30*f*, 4.103
  locating, 2.36–2.37, 2.37*f*
  outdoor spaces, 2.37–2.38, 4.35–4.36,
    4.103
  and privacy, 4.90
  policies that encourage
    personalization, 4.17–4.18
Communication
  devices, 2.87, *see also* specific types
  encouraging through furniture
    arrangement, 3.21–3.22
  with people with impaired hearing,
    1.27–1.28
  and pet therapy, 1.43
Concentration, effects of dementia on,
  2.6–2.7, 2.107–2.108
Consent, informed 3.116–3.117
Control, 4.94, 4.113
  age-related changes in, 4.98–4.100
  dementia, effects of on, 4.100–4.101
  loss of, 2.14, 2.15, 4.97, 4.97*f*
  meaningful choices, providing,
    4.105–4.107, 4.108–4.109
  perceived, 4.96
  and personality, 4.96–4.97
  policies that encourage, 4.102–4.105

  residents' regaining sense of,
    3.71–3.72
  rummaging and, 4.101
  see also Autonomy
Courtyards, access to, 2.38
Cueing systems, 2.16; *see also* Bedrooms;
  Curio cabinets; Environmental
  cues; Shadow boxes; Signage
Curio cabinets, 2.30, 2.31*f*, 3.25, 3.26*f*
Curtains, decorative, 2.176*f*

Dehydration, 2.108
Dementia, and functional disability
  cognitive factors, 2.5–2.7
  effects of on eating, 2.106, 2.107,
    2.107*f*
  environmental factors, 2.7
  feeding options in late-stage, 2.109
  and mobility, *see* Mobility
  and orientation, 2.14–2.15
  physical factors, 2.4–2.5
  and privacy needs, 4.79–4.80
  and rehabilitation, 2.52–2.53
  and relocation, *see* Relocation
  social factors, 2.7
Dentition, impact of on appetite,
  2.105–2.106, 2.105*f*
Depression, and success in physical
  rehabilitation, 2.67–2.68
De-selfing, 4.12
Diabetic retinopathy, 1.6, 1.6*t*
  overall blurred vision, 1.6
Dining rooms, 4.129–4.130
  minimize excess disability, 2.122–2.133
    carpeting, 4.132
    decor, 2.124–2.125
    furniture, 2.125–2.128, 4.130–4.132,
      4.131*f*
    lighting, 2.130–2.132, 4.132
    storage, 2.123
    subdividing rooms, 2.122–2.123,
      2.123*f*
  wayfinding, 2.35–2.36, 2.107, 2.121
Disorientation, and wandering, 3.16
  reorientation devices, 3.24–3.25
Display cases, *see* Bedrooms; Curio
  cabinets; Shadow boxes
Disrobing, inappropriate, 3.119–3.120
Disruptive behavior
  attempting to leave, *see* Attempting to
  leave

in bathing, 3.4
combative behavior, *see* Combative
  behaviors
and dementia, 3.4
during dressing, 2.157
and excess noise, 1.28–1.29
hoarding, *see* Hoarding
and music, 3.21
and privacy, threats to, *see* Combative
  behaviors
and progressively lowered stress
  threshold, 1.3
rummaging, *see* Rummaging
and scents, 1.33
socially inappropriate behaviors, *see*
  Socially inappropriate behaviors
vocalizations, *see* Vocalizations,
  disruptive
wandering, *see* Wandering
Doors
alarm/locking systems, 3.54–3.55
closet, over-the-door clothing racks,
  2.153, 2.158, 2.159*f*
knocking on before entering, staff
  approaches, 4.81–4.82, 4.102
modifications
  cognitive locks, 3.53–3.54
  dark mats, 3.52, 3.53*f*
  disguising, to minimize exiting,
    3.50, 3.51*f*
  fabric strips, 3.51, 3.52*f*
  reducing views, 3.50–3.51
    signage, 3.51–3.52, 3.54
  velvet ropes, 3.52
  wandering and, 3.28
Doorway, to bedroom
and orientation devices, 3.25, 4.27–4.28
recessed, 2.31–2.32
Double-loaded corridor floor plan,
  2.19–2.21, 2.19*f*
conversion to cluster floor plan,
  2.23–2.24, 2.24*f*
Dressing, 2.143–2.144, 2.164
ability assessment and analysis,
  2.146–2.148, 2.155
  Ws, five, 2.147–2.148
age-related changes in, 2.144–2.145
agenda behavior, 2.151–2.152
aids, 2.162–2.163
assistance, 2.146, 2.155–2.157, 2.156*f*
  gender-specific, 2.157
  residents' preferences, 4.106

Beck Dressing Performance scale,
  2.147, 2.148
closets, modifications to, 2.157–2.160
clothing
  adaptations, 2.155
  selection, 2.149–2.152
  dementia, effects of on, 2.145, 2.146,
    2.160
  dependence, levels of, 2.147*t*
  empathy with residents' difficulties,
    2.145–2.146
  grooming area, 2.161–2.162, 2.177,
    4.126, 4.127*f*
  independence, increasing, 2.152–2.153
  lighting for, improving, 2.160–2.161,
    2.161*f*
  and mobility problems, 2.155
  privacy, respecting, 2.146
  self-image tied to, 2.149–2.151
  sequencing, 2.152–2.154
  shoes, 2.155
  undressing, for bathing, 2.170
Dysphagia, 2.108–2.109

Eating, 2.103, 2.141–2.142
age-related changes, 2.104–2.106,
  2.105*f*
assisting residents, 2.115–2.116
  communication, 2.116–2.117
  residents' preferences, 4.106–4.107
creating appropriate atmosphere for,
  2.113
  administration support, 2.114
  increasing food options, 2.114
and dementia, effects of on,
  2.106–2.109, 2.112–2.113; *see also*
  Dementia, and functional
  disability
dysphagia interventions, 2.117–2.118
favorite foods, identifying, 2.111–2.112
maintaining residents' dignity, 2.119
rejecting food, 2.110–2.111
  analyzing, 2.114–2.115
utensils, adaptive, 2.133, 2.134
see also Food
Eden Alternative, 1.43, 3.72, 4.24, 4.104
Elevators, and exiting residents, 3.57–3.58
Environmental cues
for people with dementia, 2.16
encouraging use of mobility aids,
  2.62

Environmental cues—*continued*
  and purpose-specific rooms,
    4.123–4.124
  for residents of long-term care
    facilities, 2.25, 2.25*f*, 4.15–4.16
  see also specific cues
Environmental docility hypothesis, 1.2
Excess disability
  and control, 4.101
  minimizing, 2.4
    in dining, 2.120–2.133
Excessive walking, 3.10–3.11, 3.10*t*,
    3.20–3.21, 3.36
  diversions for, 3.29
  and exhaustion, 3.20–3.21
  and nutrition, 3.21
  see also Wandering
Exercise
  and falls, 2.48
  and residents with mobility problems,
    2.51–2.52, 2.65–2.67
Exiting, *see* Attempting to leave
Exposing oneself, *see* Disrobing,
    inappropriate
Expressive aphasia, 2.6

Fabrics, choosing, 4.26, 4.128
Falls, 2.47–2.48
  and bedrails, 2.81
  fears about, 2.55
  and fractures, factors influencing, 2.47
  gait changes and, 2.46
  and mobility, 2.45–2.46
  near falls, 2.55
  in people with dementia, 2.49
  preventive measures, 2.48
  and staffing patterns, 2.54–2.55
  and transfers, 2.81
Fencing
  aluminum picket, 3.47*t*
  chain link, 3.47*t*
  masonry wall, 3.47*t*
  stockade, 3.47*t*
5 Ws, *see* Ws, five
Floor plans, *see* Cluster floor plan;
    Double-loaded corridor floor
    plan; Pavilion floor plan
Floors
  and glare, 1.19, 2.74–2.76, 3.96, 3.96*f*
  and noise, treatments for, 1.29, 1.30
  nonslip, 2.69

patterned, 2.70, 2.76–2.77
resilient, 2.69, 2.70, 2.76, 2.86, 2.138,
    4.140
  versus carpeting, 2.129*t*–2.130*t*,
    4.127–4.128
sealer, 1.36
selecting, 2.76–2.77, 4.127–4.128
and shoes, 2.69–2.70
transitions, 2.76
see also Carpeting; specific rooms
Food
  accidents, handling, 2.118–2.119
  during activities, 2.120
  easily choked on, 2.118
  fanny packs, 2.108
  medical model of care and, 4.2
  puréed, 2.118
  see also Eating; Kitchens, therapeutic
Foot pain, and falls, 2.46
Front-entry bathtub, *see* Bathtubs
Functional abilities
  age-related changes in, 2.2
  assessment, 2.7–2.10
  dementia, effects of on, 2.4–2.7
  long-term care, relocating to, 2.3–2.4,
    2.10
  orientation, 2.11, 2.12
Furniture
  arrangement of
    as mobility aid, 2.70–2.71
    for privacy, 4.86
    as wandering intervention,
      3.21–3.22, 3.22*f*, 4.86
  and excess background noise,
    1.29–1.30
  institutional, and medical model of
    care, 4.12, 4.13*f*
  outdoor, 4.35–4.36
  residential-style, 2.136–2.137,
    4.135–4.136
  residents', bringing from home to
    personalize, 4.24
  wicker, choosing, 1.45
  see also specific rooms

Gait changes, age-related, and falls, 2.46
Gardening, 4.32–4.33, 4.36, 4.59–4.60
Gardens, therapeutic, 1.37–1.38, 3.46
  decorating, 4.32–4.33
  fencing for, 3.47*t*
  toxic plants, 4.163*t*–4.170*t*

Gastrointestinal problems, and appetite, 2.106
Gastrostomy tube feeding, 2.109
Glare, 1.17–1.19
  hotspots, 2.74, 2.75*f*
  reduction
    to increase mobility, 2.69
    to prevent combative behaviors, 3.95–3.97
  reflected, 2.74–2.75
Glaucoma, 1.6, 1.6*t*
  loss of peripheral vision
Gliding walker, 2.64*t*
Grab bars, 2.98, 2.99, 2.99*f*, 2.101

Hallways, 2.19, 2.20–2.21
  furniture, as mobility aid, 2.77
  handrails, 2.71–2.72, 2.77–2.78, 2.78*f*
  lighting and glare, 2.73–2.76
  and privacy, 4.87–4.88, 4.88*f*
  and scale, breaking up, 4.120, 4.121*f*
  and signage, myths about, 2.26
Handrails, 2.71–2.72, 2.77–2.78, 2.78*f*
Hearing
  age-related changes in, 1.25–1.26, 1.27–1.28
    environmental adjustments for, 1.31–1.32
    factors affecting, 1.26
  assessment, 1.27
  and dressing, problems in, 2.145
  poor
    and agnosia, 2.6
    and responses to, 1.26–1.27
Heat lamps, 2.180, 3.103
Hemiwalker, 2.64*t*
Hill-Burton Act of 1954, 4.2
History, resident's, gathering, 4.19, 4.20*f*
  and activity planning, 4.49–4.51
  privacy needs, assessing, 4.83–4.84
  Resident's Housing History form, 4.157–4.159
  Resident's Social History form, 4.147–4.156
Hoarding, 3.67–3.68, 3.71–3.72
  food, in dementia, 2.106
  see also Rummaging
Home-based philosophy of care, 4.1–4.6
  changing staff perceptions, 4.102

Hospitality model of care, 4.5–4.6
  and privacy needs, 4.79
  and residents' life roles, 4.46–4.47
Hygiene, and negative odors, 1.36; *see also* Bathing; Incontinence

Ideational apraxia, 2.147
Ideomotor apraxia, 2.147
Illuminating Engineering Society of North America, 1.15, 1.15*t*
Incontinence, 2.91
  assessing causes, 2.92–2.93
  cueing, 2.94
  and dementia, 2.92, 2.93*f*
  environmental interventions for, 2.93
  and fluid consumption, 2.95
  and immobility, 2.92
  reducing embarrassment during assistance with, 2.95–2.96
  scheduled toileting, 2.94–2.95
  sequencing cards, 2.94
Independence, promoting, as mobility aid, 2.533, 2.54
Independent activities of daily living (IADLs), 2.1
Inhibitions, lowered, 3.113–3.114
Intergenerational activities, 3.23

Kitchens, therapeutic, 2.120, 3.22, 3.23*f*, 4.58–4.59, 4.59*f*, 4.132–4.133, 4.133*f*
Knickknacks, 4.22–4.23, 4.23*f*

Lamps, residents', 4.24
Learned helplessness, 4.95
Lift-over bathtub, *see* Bathtubs
Light
  natural, benefits of, 1.7
  needs for, age-related, 1.14
  in transition areas, 1.19
Light bulbs
  and ballasts, 1.17
  and color rendering, 1.14, 1.16–1.17
Lighting, 4.138
  ambient, 1.11
    minimum levels, 1.15*t*
  can, 2.131
  chandeliers, 2.131

Lighting—*continued*
consultants, 2.84–2.85, 3.101–3.102, 2.140, 4.137–4.138
cove, 1.12, 1.16, 2.131, 2.132*f*
decorative, 4.33–4.34
diffusers, 2.73, 2.74*f*
direct, 1.12, 1.12*f*
direct down, 1.12
fluorescent, 1.14, 1.17, 4.128–4.129
and glare, 2.73–2.76, 3.96–3.97
incandescent, 1.14, 1.17
indirect, 1.11–1.13, 1.12*f*, 2.73
mobility, supporting, 2.69
night-lights, 2.79
pendant, 1.13, 1.16
poor, improving, 1.14
recessed-down, 1.12–1.13
sconce, 1.13, 2.73, 2.84, 2.132, 2.140
task, 1.13, 4.129
focused, 1.16
minimum levels, 1.16*t*
wrap-around, 2.73
see also specific rooms/areas
Locking systems, doors, 3.54–3.55
Long-term care
decor in, 4.124–4.125; *see also* specific rooms
relocating to, 2.3–2.4
and assessment of functional abilities, 2.10
and falls, 2.47
and mobility problems, 2.44
and personalization, changes in, 4.11–4.14
and role loss, 4.46
Low vision, 1.5–1.9
and agnosia, 2.6
and color cues, 2.26
and dressing aids, 2.160–2.161
and social withdrawal, 1.10

Macular degeneration, 1.6, 1.6*t*
loss of central vision, 1.6
Maintenance, regular and spot, 1.36
Massage, 1.42
Masturbation, 3.110, 3.118–3.119
Material possessions, and personalization, 4.11; *see also* Art, Furniture, Knickknacks
Mealtimes
environmental cues for, 2.35

special occasions, creating, 2.119–2.120
Medical model of care, 4.2–4.3
and privacy needs, 4.79
and residents' life roles, 4.46
Mini-Mental State Examination (MMSE), and assessing competence, 3.116
Mirrors, and impact on behavior, 3.97
MMSE, *see* Mini-Mental State Examination, and assessing competence
Mobility, 2.43–2.90
aids, 2.60–2.65, 2.83–2.84
and dementia, 2.61–2.62
furniture, 2.77
handrails, 2.71–2.72, 2.77–2.78, 2.78*f*
kinds, *see* specific types
maintaining, 2.62–2.63
praising use of, 2.61*f*
selecting, 2.62
social stigma, 2.60–2.61
and dressing, *see* Dressing
environmental adjustments for, 2.68–2.69
falls, contributors to, 2.54–2.55
goal setting to reinstate mobility, 2.57
improving, 2.72–2.76
incontinence, and immobility, 2.92
in people with dementia, 2.49–2.52
late-stage, 2.53
physiological issues, 2.45–2.48
psychological issues, 2.44
restraints, 2.57–2.58
alternatives, education about, 2.58
reducing, 2.59–2.60
use to staffing level ratio, 2.59
staff empathy, 2.56–2.57, 2.57*f*
Monitoring systems, for wandering, 3.29, 3.33–3.34, 3.56, 3.61–3.62
Mood, and sense of smell, 1.34
Multipurpose rooms, and people with dementia, 3.25–3.27, 3.27*f*
use of physical reorientation cues in, 3.27
Musculoskeletal changes, and mobility, 2.45
Music
appropriate programming, 3.94–3.95, 3.104
in bathing, 2.177
as intervention
for disruptive behavior, 3.21, 3.69
for understimulation, 3.112

Nasogastric tube feeding, 2.109
Near falls, 2.55
Neurological problems, and mobility, 2.45
Noise, background
  and people with hearing loss, 1.28
  reducing, 1.29, 3.92–3.94, 3.104
Noise Reduction Criteria, 1.30

Omnibus Budget Reconciliation Act of 1987 (PL 100-203)
  Resident's Rights section, 3.3
  and restraint use, 2.50
Orientation, 2.41–2.42
  and anxiety, 2.13
  cues, 1.21–1.22, 2.16, 4.109, 4.110*f*
  to place, 2.15–2.16
  to time, 2.15
  see also Reality orientation
Outdoor spaces
  access to by residents, 4.110
  locating/decorating, 2.37–2.38,
    4.32–4.33, 4.35–4.36
  and privacy, 4.90
  tending, residents', 4.59–4.60
Overstimulation, interventions for,
    3.86–3.87, 3.111–3.112

Pagers, 2.79
Pain, and combative behaviors, 3.78–3.79
Paint, *see* Color
Paths, 2.38
Pattern, 1.20–1.21, 2.124–2.125
Pavilion floor plan, 2.21–2.23, 2.21*f*
  conversion from racetrack plan, 2.22*f*
Perceived control, *see* Control
Personal care, providing
  and aphasia, 2.6
  discretion in, 4.82
  and impaired vision, 1.9–1.10
  and positive scents, incorporating,
    1.34–1.35
  see also Activities of daily living
Personalization, 4.37
  age-related changes in, 4.10–4.11
  "attack on self," 4.12
  decorating, 4.21
    bathrooms, 4.26–4.27
    bedrooms, 4.22–4.26, 4.27–4.29,
      4.103

common areas, 4.29–4.31
  tub room, 4.31
and dementia, effects of on, 4.14–4.16
and facilities following hospitality
    model of care, 4.12–4.13
and facilities following residential
    model of care, 4.13
outdoor spaces, 4.32–4.33, 4.35–4.36
policies that encourage, 4.17–4.18
reminiscence, 4.20–4.21
resident's history, gathering, 4.19,
    4.20*f*
self-expression, 4.7–4.8
  possessions as, 4.10–4.11, 4.13–4.14,
    4.22–4.24
self-knowledge, 4.9
"turf," 4.9
Pet therapy, 1.43, 3.113
Photographs
  as environmental cues, 2.33
  and personalization, 4.11
Physical combativeness, 3.2
Pickup walker, 2.64*t*
PL 100-203, *see* Omnibus Budget
    Reconciliation Act of 1987
PL 101-336, *see* Americans with
    Disabilities Act of 1990
Plants, 4.24, 4.104
  toxic, 4.163*t*–4.170*t*
PLST, *see* Progressively lowered stress
    threshold
Policies, facility
  control, encouraging, 4.102–4.105
  personalization, encouraging,
    4.17–4.18
  privacy, developing, 4.81–4.83
  sexual behavior, residents',
    3.114–3.115
Polypharmacy, and falls, 2.46–2.47
Preferences, residents'
  allowing, 4.103–4.104, 4.105
  in assistance with ADLs, 4.105–4.107
  and behavior tracking process, *see*
    Behavior tracking process
  documenting, 1.31, 1.35, 1.43, 1.46,
    4.49–4.51, 4.104
Presbycusis, 1.25
Privacy, 4.92
  control and, 4.107–4.108
  needs
    age-related changes in, 4.76–4.77
    dementia, effects of on, 4.79–4.80

Privacy—*continued*
    health-related changes in, 4.77–4.78
    and relocation-related changes in,
        4.78–4.79
    policies, developing, 4.81–4.83
    respecting residents', 3.85, 3.89, 4.82,
        4.83–4.85
    during bathing, 2.170, 4.82–4.83
    during dressing, 2.146
    redirecting residents infringing on
        other residents', 4.84
    spaces and times, establishing, 4.83
Progressively lowered stress threshold
    (PLST), 1.2–1.3, 3.79
Psychotropic medications, as restraints,
    2.50, 3.3
    and wandering, 3.13
Public address system, 2.79, 3.48,
    3.93–3.94
Puréed diets, 2.118

Quad cane, 2.64*t*
"Quiet areas," for overstimulated/
    agitated residents, 3.49–3.50, 3.49*f*
"Quiet times," for overstimulated/
    agitated residents, 3.87

Racetrack floor plan, 2.21–2.23, 2.22*f*; *see
    also* Double-loaded corridor floor
    plan
Reality orientation, 2.16–2.17, 3.19–3.20
Records, residents', *see* Charts, residents'
Rehabilitation, physical
    difference staff can make in success,
        2.67–2.68
    residents with dementia, 2.52–2.53
Relationships, sexual, residents' forming,
    3.109
Relocation, 2.3–2.4, 2.10, 2.44, 2.47,
    4.11–4.14
    and control, 4.99–4.100
        dementia and, 4.100–4.101
    and privacy needs, changes in,
        4.78–4.79, 4.80
    and role loss, 4.46
Reminiscence
    and personalization, encouraging,
        4.20–4.21
    photographs and, 4.11
    use of touch in, 1.42

Reminiscing art, *see* Art
Repetitive behavior, 3.110–3.111, 3.121
    interventions for, 3.120
    and therapeutic touch, 1.42
Residential character, in long-term care
    settings, creating, 4.115–4.141
Residential model of care, 4.3–4.5
    and residents' life roles, 4.47
Residents' council, 4.105
Resident's Housing History form,
    4.157–4.159
Resident's Social History form,
    4.147–4.156
Resistance to care, *see* Combative
    behaviors
Restraints, 2.50–2.51, 2.57–2.58, 3.2–3.3
    alternatives to, 2.58, 3.3
    associated behaviors, 2.51, 3.12
    BASs, 2.82
    reducing, 2.59–2.60
    removal, preparing residents for,
        2.59–2.60
    subtle forms, 3.13
    use to staffing level ratio, 2.59
Roles, as self-definition, 4.40–4.41
    dementia, effects of on, 4.47–4.48
    domestic activities and, 4.52–4.53
    leisure activities and, 4.42–4.43,
        4.53–4.54
    offstage, 4.71–4.73
        and control, sense of, 4.73–4.74
        self-protection, 4.74–4.76
        self-reflection, 4.73
    role confusion, 4.45
    role loss, 4.41
        life changes and, 4.43–4.44
        physical changes, 4.44
        and search for new roles, 4.45
    as self-worth measure, 4.41–4.42
    work activities and, 4.53
    see also Activities; Privacy; Relocation
Rolling walker, 2.64*t*
Room dividers, 2.123, 2.134–2.135, 4.134
    for privacy, 4.89
    and scale, 4.118, 4.120–4.122
Roommate pairing process, involving
    residents in, 4.104–4.105
Rooms, purpose-specific, 4.122–4.124
Routines, residents', importance of
    preserving and using, 3.85–3.86
Rummaging, 3.65
    and control, *see* Control

creating areas for, 3.68–3.69, 3.70, 3.72
  rummaging drawers, 3.29, 3.70
  sensory stimulation boards, 3.71
  "workplaces," 3.71
environmental adjustments for, 3.74
and interfering with others, 3.70
  redirecting, 4.84
needing to feel productive and,
  3.66–3.67, 3.69
and privacy, 4.80
stimulation, increasing, 3.69
triggers, 3.65
and wandering, 3.10
see also Hoarding

Safe Return, 3.45, 3.58
Safety, and residents with dementia,
  2.50–2.53
Scolding, ineffectiveness of, 3.114
Sensory cues, see Hearing; Smell (sense
  of); Taste, age-related changes in;
  Touch; Vision
Sensory impairments, 1.1
  and cognitive impairment, 1.2
  and mobility, 2.45
Sensory Stimulation Assessment form,
  3.133–3.134
  use of, 3.48, 3.92, 3.131–3.132
Sensory stimuli, 1.1
  and activities for people with
    dementia, 1.3
  conflicting, 1.3–1.4
  and hallucinations, 1.3
  impact on people with dementia,
    1.2–1.3
  quality of, 1.3
  tactile stimulation, importance of,
    3.66, 3.67f, 3.113
  special napkins, 3.72
Sequencing cards, 2.94, 2.100, 3.86
  dressing, 2.153–2.154, 2.162
Sexual advances, 3.119
Sexual behaviors, residents'
  between residents, 3.116–3.117
  between residents and nonresidents,
    3.115–3.116
  facility policies, 3.114–3.115
  inappropriate, 3.107–3.110, 3.117–3.120
  staff training, 3.115, 3.121, 3.122
  see also Consent, informed
Sexually ambiguous behavior, 3.110

Shadow boxes, 2.40, 3.25, 3.33
Shadowing, 3.40
Shelving, 4.22–4.23, 4.23f, 4.162, 4.162f
Shoes
  dressing, 2.155
  effective for mobility, 2.69–2.70
Showering, 2.175
  shower curtains, half height, 2.175,
    2.179, 3.89, 3.99
  shower manufacturers, 2.178–2.179
  shower wands, hand-held, 2.175, 3.88,
    3.89f
  see also Bathing
Side-entry bathtub with door, see
  Bathtubs
Side-entry tilting bathtub, see Bathtubs
Signage
  appropriate, 2.39–2.40, 3.32–3.33,
    3.60–3.61
  as detour cue, 3.28
  directional, 2.25f, 2.34f, 2.100
  and hazardous areas, 3.28
  and lighting, 2.26
  placement, 2.27–2.28
  as reorientation device, 3.25
  inappropriate, 2.27f
Single-tipped cane, 2.64t
Skin care, 1.41
Slide transfer benches, 2.175, 2.179
Smell (sense of)
  age-related changes in, 1.33
  environmental adjustments for, 1.39
  aromatherapy, 1.37
  food as a sensory cue, 1.37
  and personal care, see Personal care,
    providing
Socially inappropriate behaviors,
  3.105–3.122
Spa model of care, see Hospitality model
  of care
Spatial adjacencies, 2.18–2.19
  cluster floor plan, 2.23–2.24
  double-loaded corridors, 2.19–2.21,
    2.19f, 2.20f
  pavilion floor plan, 2.21–2.23
  and residential character in long-term
    care facilities, 4.116–4.118, 4.118f,
    4.119f
Staffing patterns, 2.54–2.55
Stimulation
  limiting, 3.48
  providing, 3.45–3.46, 3.46f

Stimulation—*continued*
  Sensory Stimulation Assessment,
    3.48, 3.133
  see also Sensory stimuli
Stress incontinence, 2.91
Sundowning syndrome, minimizing, 1.7,
    1.19

Tables, dining, 2.126–2.128, 2.127*f*, 2.135
  adjustable-height, 4.134, 4.139
Tags, for wandering residents,
    3.56–3.57
Taste, age-related changes in, 1.33–1.34
Telephone usage, 4.104
Television programming, 3.94, 3.104
Temperature regulation, 1.45, 4.103
  thermostats, 4.111
Tense perseverance, 3.111
Texture, importance of in environment,
    1.44
  as an orientation cue, 1.44
Toilet
  locating, by residents with dementia,
    2.35, 2.96–2.98, 2.97*f*
  seats, distinguished by color, 2.100
Toileting
  and falls in people with dementia,
    2.49
  privacy, protecting residents' during,
    4.84–4.85
  reducing embarrassment during
    assistance with, 2.95–2.96
  scheduled, 2.94–2.95
  sequencing cards and, 2.94, 2.100
  Behavior Tracking Form, 2.94,
    3.127–3.129
  see also Incontinence
Touch
  age-related changes in, 1.41–1.42
  environmental adjustments for,
    1.44, 1.46
  appropriate, 3.119
  inappropriate, 1.43, 3.119
  skin care, 1.41
  therapeutic, 1.41–1.42
Towel bath, 2.169–2.170
Toys, appropriateness for older adults,
    1.43
Transfers, 2.81
  slide transfer benches, 2.175, 2.179
  to and from toilet, 2.98–2.100

Tub rooms
  creating pleasant atmosphere in,
    2.176–2.177, 2.176*f*, 3.92, 3.93*f*
  creating privacy in, 2.171, 2.171*f*, 4.89
  decorating, 4.31, 4.129, 4.130*f*
  temperature, controlling, 2.172,
    2.175–2.176
  see also Bathtubs

Understimulation, interventions for,
    3.111–3.112
Undressing
  for bathing, 2.170
  preventing combative behaviors, 3.84
  see also Bathing; Dressing
Urge incontinence, 2.91

Validation, versus reality orientation,
    2.16–2.17
Verbal combativeness, 3.2
Vision
  age-related changes in, 1.5–1.9, 1.23
  environmental adjustments for,
    1.23–1.24
  dementia and, 1.7, 1.8*f*, 1.9
  low, *see* Low vision
  shadows and, 1.15–1.16
Visual cliffing, 2.70, 2.71*f*
Visuospatial dysfunction, and agnosia,
    2.14
Vocalizations, disruptive
  assessing, 3.106–3.107
  staff interventions, 3.111–3.114
  and understimulation, 3.112–3.113
  staff's influence, 3.107
  triggers, 3.105–3.106, 3.106*t*, 3.107,
    3.113–3.114
  understanding, 3.107, 3.121, 3.122

Ws, five, 2.72, 2.114–2.115, 4.51, 4.106
  and Beck Dressing Performance scale,
    2.147
Walkers, 2.63–2.65, 2.64*t*
Walking clubs, 3.18
Wall decor
  for dining areas, 2.128, 2.130
  as reorientation device, 2.19–2.20,
    3.24–3.25
  selecting, as mobility aid, 2.76–2.77

Wandering, 3.1, 3.9–3.11, 3.10*t*,
    3.36–3.37
  activity programming, 3.29–3.31, 3.36
  and agenda behavior, 3.4
  and agenda behavior approach,
    3.14–3.15, 3.15*f*
  and disorientation, 3.16
    cues to reorientation, 3.20
  environmental adjustments for,
    3.21–3.29
  excessive walking, *see* Excessive walking
  and furniture as intervention,
    3.21–3.22, 3.22*f*, 4.86
  limiting, 3.28–3.29
  monitoring systems, 3.29, 3.33–3.34,
    3.56, 3.61–3.62
  motivators for, 3.11, 3.12*t*
  and nonwanderers, differences
    between, 3.11
  perceptions about, 3.21
  and programming, 3.15–3.16
    engaging previous interests,
    3.16–3.18
    structured activities, 3.18–3.19
  and reality orientation, 3.19–3.20
  and redirection, 3.13–3.14, 3.14*f*,
    3.36
  and resident's anxiety, 3.16
  and restraints, 3.12
Water, and bathing, 2.172, 2.175; *see also*
    Bathing

Wayfinding, and orientation, 2.11–2.12,
    2.13
  dementia and, 2.14, 2.16, 2.18; *see also*
    Color; Signage; Spatial
    adjacencies
  see also specific rooms
Wealshire, The, 4.117–4.118, 4.119*f*
Well-being, feelings of, 4.95–4.97
Wheelchairs, 2.65
Windows
  and excess noise, treatments for, 1.29
  and exiting residents, 3.58
  and glare, 1.18, 2.74
    blinds, 1.18–1.19, 3.95
    reducing, to prevent combative
    behaviors, 3.95–3.97
  treatments, bedroom, 4.28–4.29
  and ventilation, residents' control
    over, 4.103
Withdrawal, social
  and diminishment of functional
    abilities, 2.1–2.2
  dementia, 2.7
  mobility problems, 2.44
  orientation problems, 2.13
  and low vision, 1.10
  and threats to privacy needs, 4.79
Work life roles, and activities planning,
    4.53
  creating workplaces, 4.60
  workshops, 4.61–4.62, 4.61*f*

ORDER THESE COMPANION VIDEOS FOR CREATING SUCCESSFUL DEMENTIA CARE SETTINGS

Video 1
Maximizing Cognitive and Functional Abilities/No. 2769/40-min VHS/$92

Video 2
Minimizing Disruptive Behaviors/No. 2777/21-min VHS/$55

Video 3
Enhancing Self and Sense of Home/No. 2785/33-min VHS/$78

Prices are subject to change.

ORDER FORM

Please send me the following video(s):

Stk No.	Title	Quantity	Price

SHIPPING & HANDLING				
For pre-tax total of	*Add*	Subtotal		
$0.00 to $49.99	$5.00	MD residents, add 5% tax		
$50.00 to $399.99	10%	Shipping & Handling		
$400.00 and over	8%	TOTAL		

❑ Check enclosed (payable to **Health Professions Press**)
❑ Bill my institution (attach purchase order) ❑ MasterCard ❑ Visa ❑ AmEx

Credit card#/Exp. date _____

Signature _____

Name _____

Address _____
(Orders cannot be shipped to P.O. boxes)
City/State/ZIP _____

Daytime phone _____

HEALTH PROFESSIONS PRESS P.O. BOX 10624 BALTIMORE, MD 21285-0624
TOLL FREE (888) 337-8808   FAX (410) 337-8539
www.healthpropress.com

ZCK